Dental Health Education

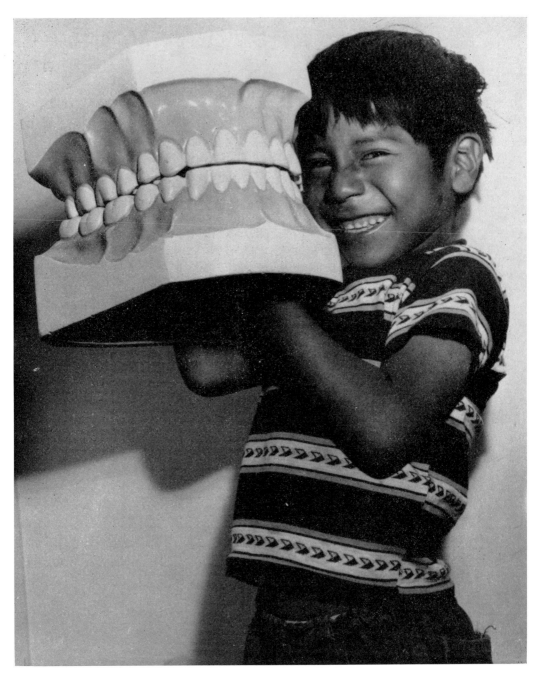

Little Indians learn about dental health. (Courtesy, Indian Health Service, Dental Branch, U. S. Public Health Service, Department of Health, Education and Welfare.)

Dental Health Education

FOR THE
EDUCATION OF INDIVIDUALS DURING DENTAL TREATMENT,
SCHOOL DENTAL HEALTH PROGRAMS
AND IN PUBLIC HEALTH PROGRAMS

FRANCES A. STOLL, R.D.H., Ed.D.
Professor Emeritus, Columbia University

JOAN L. CATHERMAN, R.D.H., M.S.
*Director of Dental Hygiene Education, Council of Dental Education,
American Dental Association*

FOURTH EDITION, *Thoroughly Revised*

Illustrated

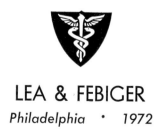

LEA & FEBIGER
Philadelphia · 1972

ISBN 0–8121–0386–6

Library of Congress Catalog Card Number 70-152031

Published in Great Britain by Henry Kimpton Publishers, London

PRINTED IN THE UNITED STATES OF AMERICA

DEDICATED TO THE MEMORY OF

HAROLD PAUL STOLL

WHO MADE ALL THE EDITIONS POSSIBLE

Preface

Knowledge is of two kinds. We know a subject ourselves or we know where we can find information upon it.

Samuel Johnson

The fourth edition of *Dental Health Education* is new in all respects. Before the preparation of the manuscript, the authors surveyed the instructors of all the schools of dental hygiene to learn their ideas about how the book might be more useful. Many of their recommendations, suggestions and information have been included and give the book its broad scope.

This edition of *Dental Health Education*, like its predecessors, is written primarily for dental hygienists, who are required in all types of practice to be accomplished health educators. Many of the original ideas in the book have evolved from the authors' teaching experiences in public schools; from private office practice and from their wide experience in educating dental hygienists and in supervising and instructing dental hygiene teachers. It is a text which can be used in a number of courses required by accreditation organizations and the National Board Examinations. Students and teachers will find it useful for the dental health education aspects of pre-clinical dental hygiene, clinical practice and office management. It should prove an especially valuable adjunct in preparing students and instructors for intern-teaching and supervision.

This edition of *Dental Health Education* will also be useful for public health educators who find a dearth of scientific information on dental health in general texts on health. It contains new information regarding such topics as dental health insurance plans, incremental dental treatment for children and reports and statistics about community health programs. Classroom teachers will find a wealth of information about lesson plans and source materials as well as suggested projects to encourage realistic participation by pupils. Administrators faced with the problems of instituting new school dental health programs will find data about standards of instruction, service and treatment in the text. The bibliographies of preceding editions have been replaced by lists of Selected Readings which provide the most recent literature in research and theory in dental health. New schools of dental hygiene and their teachers will be able to use these lists to build a reference library of periodicals, journals and texts pertaining to dental health and educational method.

The concept of health education in this edition of *Dental Health Education* was formulated by the "School Health Education Study," which was conducted on a grant from the Bronfman Foundation and supported by the National Education Association, the U.S. Office of Education, the U.S. Public Health Service and the National Congress of Parents and Teachers. This study concluded that dental health is a vital part of personal hygiene and community health. Some of the findings of the study were that,

> Only one of five students at the sixth grade level brushed or rinsed their mouth regularly after eating.
> Students' knowledge and attitudes about health in the ninth grade were considerably better than their health practices.
> Only one in two of the ninth grade group could identify the recommended method for brushing the teeth.

Instructional problems that were reported by the study indicate that the following conditions exist:

> failure of the home to encourage practice of health learned in school
> insufficient time in the school day for health instruction
> ineffectiveness of instruction method
> inadequate professional preparation of staff
> failure of parents to follow up on needed and recommended health services for children
> indifference toward health education on the part of teachers, parents, administrators and health officers in the community, hence, student indifference to health education

These facts emphasize that dental health instruction is vital in order to provide our children with scientific knowledge so that they can develop good health habits that will serve them throughout life. The purpose of the fourth edition of *Dental Health Education*, then, is to enhance the effectiveness of instruction of dental health concepts.

The authors are indebted to the directors, instructors and students of all the dental hygiene schools that participated in the survey that preceded the writing of this text. We wish to express particular thanks to Louise Ciora, R.D.H., Chief of the Dental Division of the Commonwealth of Pennsylvania, for her cooperation in updating the dental health program of that state. We are also indebted to the American Dental Association for the privilege of using some of their visual materials; the Indian Health Service, Dental Branch, Department of Health, Education and Welfare, for the fine illustrations on dental health; numerous professional associations for their aid in providing reprints, statistics and other important information; and to the commercial companies who provided illustrations. All have helped to make this text unique in dental health literature; it remains the only book-length text on the subject of education for dental health.

Frances A. Stoll, Ed. D.
Winter Park, Florida

Joan L. Catherman, M.S.
Chicago, Illinois

Contents

Chapter 4. *Opportunities for Individual Instruction During Dental Treatment*

Chapter 5. *Dental Disease—A Public Health Problem*

Chapter 6. *Dental Treatment for All Children*

Chapter 7. *Preventive Measures for Dental Health*

Chapter 8. *The Community Dental Health Program*

INTRODUCTION TO DENTAL HEALTH EDUCATION

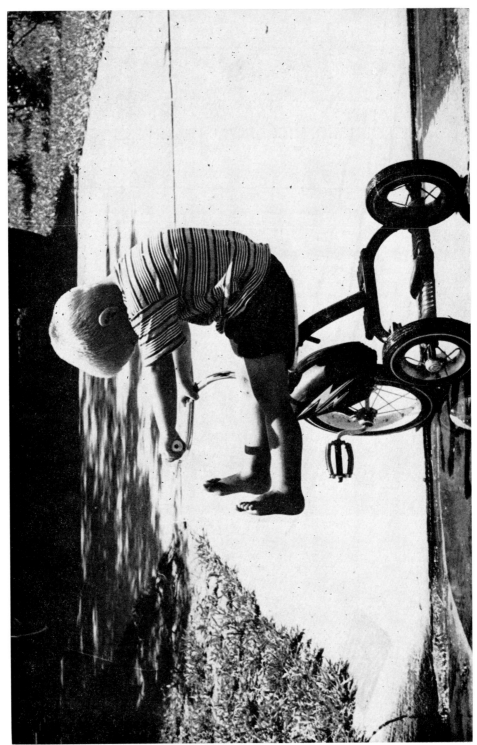

Fig. 1.—At three years of age, Jimmy brushes his own teeth, goes to the dentist and rides a tricycle. (Courtesy, Orlando Sentinel, Orlando, Florida.)

Chapter 1

Foundations of Dental Health Education

What is Health?

The history of man's fight for health begins with what little is known about his earliest existence when he was completely at the mercy of nature with no effective means of combating its hazards. Then came the slow process of learning that occupied man for centuries as he advanced in civilization. He learned that technology could raise his standard of living, improve his health and increase his longevity. Research in medical and dental sciences has resulted in a dramatic acceleration in health knowledge. In this increasingly complex twentieth century, knowledge is growing at an unprecedented rate. Consequently, reassessment of health goals has been intensified and the search goes on for ways of developing each individual so that he will assume a responsible role in society and find added satisfaction in living.

Health is not merely the absence of disease and illness; it is a state of complete physical, mental and social well-being. The trend in health education is toward increased emphasis on prevention and the acceptance of the idea that health involves a positive factor. It is necessary to do more than cure disease in order to maintain good health. Health knowledge contributes to good health, but unless attitudes and habits are developed and put into practice, little will be gained.

Normal functioning of all parts of the body contributes to one's ability to do a full day's work without undue fatigue. Normal function also increases enthusiasm for living, cheerfulness, attractiveness and self-esteem. Conversely, mental and social well-being contributes to physical health. Fortunately, Americans are health-conscious; they are continuously searching for ways to better health.

What is Health Education?

Health education is the result of the efforts made on the part of an organized society to help people learn to live healthfully. This education may take place in the home, in the school or in the community and it may occur during work hours or during leisure time. Its *content* is largely derived from medicine, public health and physical, biological and social sciences. The full scope of health education covers many diverse areas, one of which is dental health. Health problems and their solutions need to be presented in an integrated and meaningful way so that the learner sees the biological, social, cultural, economic and political implications of his actions in reference to health matters.

Health knowledge must be broadened to include an understanding of the individual's responsibility in helping to solve family, community, national and world health problems. A more knowledgeable adult population should be the result of these wider concepts. This generation should be aware of and competent to deal with current health problems and those of future generations as health education reaches larger segments of the population.

When a child enters school, he has many attitudes and health practices which have been acquired at home. Some of these may not be scientifically sound and may need modification; some must be reinforced. Effective changes in an individual's health behavior should be related to personal goals, attitudes and values. Changes in health behavior are affected by group mores, socioeconomic background, and environmental pressures.

The *methodology* of health education is derived largely from the behavioral sciences, particularly sociology and psychology. The individuality of the learner and the learning process are of paramount importance. Learning does not take place unless the individual is actively involved in the process. The participation may be physical, mental or emotional. Health education personnel seek to help the individual discover his problems and take action in solving them.

Relevance of Health Education in the Total Population

In a recently published study conducted from 1941 to 1962, interesting patterns of public knowledge regarding health and illness emerged. It was found that health knowledge rises with increased education. A national sample of the population was asked if they knew the purpose of adding fluorides to drinking water. Those who were able to identify the purpose of the fluoride ranged from less than high school education, 28% to college graduates, 81%.

The results of the study also indicated that health knowledge rises with income and occupational status. It tends to be inversely related to age because the younger generation has received more health instruction than those over sixty years of age. Women seem to have better health knowledge than men, namely because women feel more responsibility for the family health. Printed materials are more likely than television to be a source of public knowledge of health. More people reported that they obtained health information more from reading than from seeing television programs on health.*

Health education is a unity of man's physical, mental and social well-being resulting from informed judgement.

Health behavior is based on knowledge, attitudes and practices.

The focus of health education is the individual, the family, and the community, in that order.

All the components are interdependent and result in dynamic interaction.

Concepts of Health Education

Within the last five years, there has been a decided change of thought concerning the content and method used in teaching health. The School Health Education Study of 1964-1965 uses the "Key Concepts" idea as the goal toward which learning should be directed in health education from kindergarten through grade twelve. These key concepts are identified as:

A. *Growing and Developing*
Concepts: 1. Body structure and function influences growth and development and vice versa.
2. Growth and development follows a predictable sequence, yet is unique for each individual.

B. *Decision Making*
Concepts: 1. Personal health practices, including dental health, are affected by a complexity of sources which are often conflicting.
2. Use of health information, products and services is governed by the application of an individual's criteria.
3. Use of stimulants and depressants arises from a variety of motivations.
4. Food selection and eating

---

* Wade, S.: "Public Knowledge about Health," *American Journal of Public Health*, March, 1970, p. 485.

patterns are determined by physical, mental, social, cultural and economic factors.

C. Interactions

Concepts: 1. Protection and promotion of health are an individual, a family and a community concern.

2. Whatever the environment, the potential for hazards and accidents exists.

3. There is a reciprocal relationship between man, disease and environment.

4. The family is the basic unit of society through which certain health needs can be fulfilled.

These concepts are not considered as separate or unrelated areas of study; rather, they are interdependent and inter-related to one another.*

Concepts expressed in a more formal type of study pattern have been stated as health values:†

1. The relation between knowledge and health
2. Health values
3. Health progress and problems
4. Health potential
5. Health appraisal

No matter which approach in the educative process is used, health education personnel accept the individual as he is and seek to help him find more healthful ways of living.

Dental Health, A Major Area of Health Education

Dental disease is said to be pandemic at all times. As yet, no infallible *cures* have been discovered. Work is progressing toward better means of prevention through research. Dental health education for parents and children has proved to be the most promising approach to the problems of dental disease. Protection from infection of the dental structures depends largely on mouth hygiene, most of which is performed in the home.

Teeth are not indispensable structures. Nevertheless, there are good physiological, sociological and psychological reasons for prizing our teeth and deploring their premature loss.

Up to 98% of children will at some time in their school lives experience tooth decay, disease of the supporting tissues or other deviations from normal dental health. The margin of safety for teeth is narrow compared with many other body structures; further, there is inadequate provision for self-repair. Thus, preventive measures taken early in life are particularly valuable in saving teeth for a lifetime of usefulness.

That dental health education is effective in reducing dental disease is indicated by a recent survey of dental services rendered in 1969. The survey states:

Of the 35,783 patients included in this nation-wide survey more than 25% were between 10 and 19 years of age. The dental services received by the greatest number of patients were oral examinations, prophylaxis, radiographs, one and two surface amalgam fillings. These treatments are classed as *preventive services.*

The survey indicates that significant changes have occurred in the proportion of patients receiving various services since similar surveys were conducted in 1950 and 1959. The percentage of patients receiving extractions, fillings and dentures has declined while there is an increase in the percentage of patients receiving prophylaxis, radiographic examinations, fluoride treatments and orthodontic corrections.‡

It is reasonable to believe that the improvement shown in the survey can be attributed to increased knowledge concerning dental health, particularly among the private dental office patients.

---

* The curriculum phase of SCHOOL HEALTH EDUCATION STUDY: A SUMMARY REPORT, 1964, as reported by Fodor and Dalis, HEALTH INSTRUCTION: THEORY AND APPLICATION, Lea & Febiger, Philadelphia, 1966.

† Turner, C. E.: PERSONAL AND COMMUNITY HEALTH. 13th. Edition, Mosby Co., St. Louis, 1967, p. 5.

‡ Moen, B. D., Poetsch, F. E.: "More Preventive Care, Less Tooth Repair," Journal American Dental Association, July, 1970, p. 25.

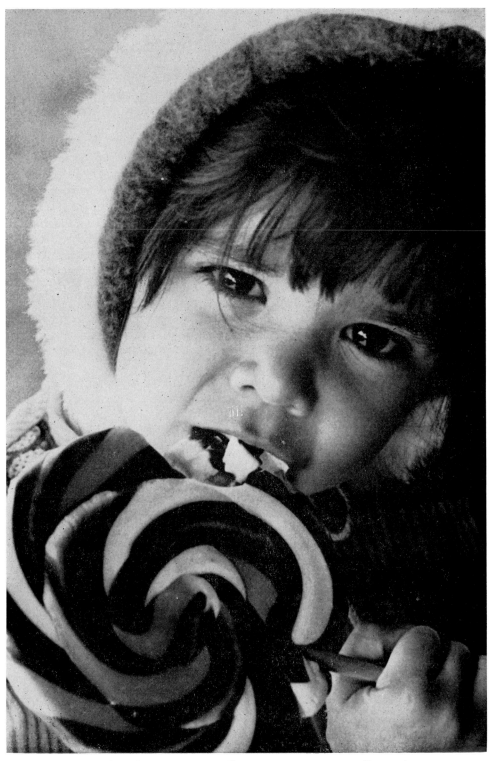

FIG. 2.—Newspaper heading, "Betty Has Her Lollipop To Keep Her Warm." But what is happening to her teeth? (Courtesy, Orlando Sentinel, Orlando, Florida.)

Chapter 2

The Significance of Dental Health
to Total Health

Dental information is penetrating the wall of ignorance and misunderstanding in regard to dental disease in only 25% of the population. These are the people who are convinced that dental neglect has a deleterious effect on general well-being. Dental defects and disease are accumulating in the rest of the population six times faster than they are being treated.

Dental Caries

The disease which produces cavities in teeth is known as dental caries. It is unquestionably the most prevalent dental disease among children between the ages of three and eighteen. The first lesions may appear soon after the eruption of the first teeth. Pits and fissures in tooth surfaces are more susceptible than the smooth surfaces. The chewing surfaces of the molar teeth seem to be attacked first. Girls seem to be slightly more susceptible to such attacks than boys, probably because girls' teeth erupt earlier and are therefore exposed longer to the ravages of decay.

Dental plaque, a highly acid, gelatinous substance that adheres to the teeth, causes decalcification of tooth enamel and appears to be the leading factor in tooth decay. Lactobacillus and certain strains of streptococci have been found in the dental plaque and appear to be the producers of the acid-forming enzymes. While the exact nature of dental plaque is not known, there is evidence that it is a protein substance formed from saliva in the form of mucin. As this substance traps microorganisms, it grows into a dense matted mass.

Acute Infections of the Mucosa

The diseases in this group are transitory and may recur from time to time. Most of the simple inflammatory diseases in children, known as *gingivitis*, are due to accumulations of food debris and poor toothbrushing technique. The best control is supervised brushing, regular prophylaxis and brushing directly after eating.

Herpes simplex, known as "fever sores," is seen in both children and adults. It is caused by a virus which remains in the soft tissues of the mouth long after the acute stage is over and it may recur from time to time if the individual's resistance is lowered. The onset of herpes may be very severe, with high temperature and general disability. The entire mouth and throat may be highly inflamed. The disease tends to "cure itself," and no particular treatment is prescribed. Herpes is infectious and may become epidemic in schools. The secondary lesion appears on the lips and is known as "cold sores"; if the lesion is in the mouth, as "canker sores."

Vincent's infection is a serious acute infection of the gingiva which tends to become chronic. It is a disease brought on by lowered resistance of the individual. It is caused by a pathogenic bacteria but is not considered communicable. It responds to a thorough cleaning of the teeth which removes all calculus and debris. A strict regimen of mouth hygiene must be observed consistently. Individuals who have Vincent's infection should have a thorough physical examination to determine the cause of low vitality.

The simplest gingival irritation should be regarded as a condition which may lead to more serious periodontal disturbance. The individual should remain under dental observation at regular intervals.

Periodontal Diseases

Periodontal disease is actually a group of diseases affecting the supporting tissues of the teeth. They are the most common cause of tooth loss in adult life. Periodontal disease is now recognized as a public health problem because of the number of persons affected, and as such, it must receive greater emphasis both in the educational phase and in prevention and cure. Periodontal disease affects the bony structures and the soft tissues surrounding the teeth. The onset of the disease is being recognized more frequently among children than in the past.

Because of the involvement of several types of tissues in periodontal disease, no one causative factor can be stated. There seem to be two sets of predisposing factors: (a) local diseased conditions in the mouth, and (b) systemic disease. The best prevention is correction of local conditions such as complete systematic removal of all dental calculus, plaque and debris; and correction of all irritating force upon the tissues such as cavities, poor restorations, abnormal occlusion and mouth habits.

The systemic factors that predispose to periodontal disease are malnutrition, vitamin deficiencies, debilitating diseases such as tuberculosis, kidney disease, virus infections, allergies and psychic disturbances.

Recently it was found that smoking was directly related to a higher prevalence of periodontal disease.

Malocclusion and Congenital Deformities

The entire form and function of the face and jaws are directly affected and governed by the manner in which the teeth of the upper jaw meet and fit with the teeth of the lower jaw. The exact pattern of closure is termed occlusion, which is further defined as the space relation between the teeth in the action of closing and chewing (see the Appendix).

The establishment of the occlusion of the teeth begins at about six months of age and ends with the eruption of the third molars. More accurately, the development of occlusion is a long and constantly changing process beginning with conception and extending throughout life.

Malocclusion is any deviation from the normal pattern of occlusion. It tends to impair masticatory function; to increase susceptibility to dental caries; to predispose toward periodontal disease; to lead to the early loss of teeth and abnormal respiratory habits; to provoke abnormal mental attitudes in relation to facial esthetics; and to impair speech.

Function is an important factor in the continued growth and development of the human body. In addition to function, growth is appreciably affected by many other factors, including heredity, environment, nutrition and general health. Prevention and correction of malocclusion are important factors in the growth and development of the whole child and as such deserve due consideration in the health program of the school and the community.

There are many forms of facial deformities including cleft palate that must be considered as dental health problems affecting the total well-being of the individual. Due consideration should be given to all abnormalities of the mouth and teeth as they affect the total health of the child.

Neuropsychic Effect of Poorly Formed Teeth and Jaws

An important phase of dental health frequently ignored is the neuropsychic effect of poorly formed, decayed teeth upon the social behavior of children. There is increasing evidence that dentists, psychiatrists and others interested in the emotional development of children are paying heed to the effect of bad teeth, particularly in the age of adolescence. These are important years in social development and adjustment, during which boys and girls become acutely aware of social pressures and relationships. The opinions and attitudes of peers have a deep influence on an adolescent's feeling of acceptance or rejection.

Any deviation in dress, appearance or manner from the mode of the group is actually painful to the child. The individual who does not conform is open to ridicule. Recognizing these factors, one can readily understand the significance of "ugly teeth." Personal appearance affects social status within the group and sets a child apart from those with whom he is trying to form close relationships. Conflicts develop, as in the case of the fourteen-year-old who refuses to continue school because she has "crooked teeth" or in the case of boys dating only the pretty girls. Another example is the girl of thirteen who refuses dental treatment because she is ashamed to show her teeth to the dentist.

Other emotional maladjustments are indicated by habits involving the teeth and the mouth. Thumb-sucking, while normal in the very young child, usually stops when the physiological desire to suck is satisfied. If discontinued at an early age, it does not cause malocclusion. But when the habit continues for several years longer, malocclusion results and the reason why the child continues thumb-sucking should be investigated. He may be unable to progress normally with solutions to his problems so he resorts to an earlier form of gratification to relieve his tension. In this category are also such habits as nail biting, lip sucking and tongue thrust.

Speech Problems

The more commonplace defects are often overlooked in considering the more dramatic dental conditions. Most children learn to talk without much help, but some acquire undesirable habits during the learning period. Some of the problems of faulty speech are directly connected with dysfunction, malformation or pernicious habits involving the tongue, teeth, throat and lips. The same structures are used in speaking as are used in breathing, sucking, swallowing, chewing, and coughing.

The dental phase of speech correction pertains to the recognition and correction of all defects in the mouth and teeth. It also includes the education of the parents and child concerning the undesirable habit so that proper treatment may be started before the habit becomes fixed or the structures of the mouth and teeth damaged.

Diet and Nutrition in Relation to Dental Health

It has been shown through a number of studies that man does not meet his nutritional needs on the basis of appetite or custom. Appetite is not a reliable guide to the selection of an adequate diet. Refining, processing, and cooking often appeal to the palate at the sacrifice of vital food factors including minerals and vitamins.

Calcium and phosphorus are the two elements found in the hard structures of teeth (dentin and enamel) along with traces of a number of other minerals. These nutrients are procured principally from high protein foods, fruits and vegetables and are deposited in the teeth with the aid of vitamins.

The main dietary factor affecting teeth in their formative stages that makes them resistant to decay is fluoride. There are rarely sufficient fluorides found in food to build decay-resistant teeth so that it must be supplied in some other form. The most economical method is the addition of fluoride to drinking water. Masses of people are benefited by the addition of 1ppm (1 part per million) of fluoride to communal water supplies. This topic is discussed at length in Chapter 7, Preventive Measures for Dental Health.

Free sugars and fermentable carbohydrates lodged on the teeth for even a short period of time, ten or fifteen minutes, will result in the formation of acid which causes tooth decay. A reduction in the *frequency* of intake is more important than the amount consumed as far as dental decay is concerned. Each fresh supply of sugar is an additional attack on the teeth.

Dietary deficiencies affect the health of the gingival tissues and the periodontal tissues surrounding the teeth. The lack of vitamin C produces a gingivitis which in its most acute form extends to the periodontal membranes. Deficiencies of vitamin C lead to the lack of collagen, an important protein substance found in connective tissue, cartilage and bone. Lack of collagen is seen as swollen, bleeding gingiva.

Research indicates that there is a direct relationship between the physical character of diet and the health of the soft tissues and bone supporting the teeth. Stimulation derived from strenuous chewing of tough fibrous foods causes an increase in the circulation of the blood and the consequent improvement in the "tone" of the tissues, just as exercise improves the tone of muscles. Diets which lack sufficient hard foods that require strenuous chewing will reduce the functional demand on the supporting bone and cause atrophy of the dental structures due to disuse.

Detergent foods such as tough meats, hard breads and raw vegetables and fruits that require considerable chewing also tend to retard the development of calculus on teeth. Civilized man must consume a diet that is not only adequate in nutrients, vitamins and minerals but also one that contains sufficient hard detergent foods to require considerable chewing.

The dental health problem is a complex one. It has been demonstrated that dental health or the lack of it affects all phases of child development and all areas of his environment, school, home and community. Neglect of any area of dental health results in far-reaching effects on the growth and development of the individual.

Questions for Review and Discussion

1. Describe the process of tooth decay so that it can be understood by a sixth-grade child.

2. State the conditions that might be found in the mouth of a child that would indicate the onset of periodontal disease.

3. Upon what evidence can periodontal disease be considered a public health problem?

4. Which disease causes greater loss of teeth: (a) dental caries, (b) periodontal disease? 1. in childhood, 2. in adults?

5. Define a pernicious habit. Name several that might affect the health of the mouth and teeth.

6. Adequate diet is considered essential to normal health. Teeth are affected by poor diet. Convince a group of teen-agers that sugar drinks, candy and hot dogs do not constitute a good diet.

7. What role does vitamin C play in dental health?

8. Mastication is the process of chewing food. Name the physiological conditions that affect mastication.

9. What factors of diet increase the health of the dental structures?

10. Correction of local conditions in the mouth is the best prevention known for periodontal disease. Name some local conditions which predispose an individual toward periodontal disease.

11. Discuss the importance of sound teeth in a clean mouth in relation to good mental health.

12. In your clinical experience observe and bring to class for discussion examples of poor mental health that might be connected with dental disorders.

Selected Readings

Christensen, G. J.: "Research in Clinical Dentistry —Prevalence of Periodontal Disease," Journal American Dental Association, September, 1969, p. 676.

Haryett, R. D., Hansen, F. C., Sandlands, M. L.: "Chronic Thumbsucking, the Psychological Effects and the Relative Effectiveness of Various Methods of Treatment," American Journal of Orthodontics, August, 1967, p. 563.

Miller, H.: "Treatment Procedure for Early Occlusal Disharmonies Caused by Noxious Habits," Journal American Dental Association, August, 1969, p. 361.

Sharp, G. S., Helsper, J. T.: "Oral Manifestations of Systemic Disease," Journal Oral Surgery, Oral Medicine and Oral Pathology, June, 1967, p. 737.

Soloman, H. A., Priore, R. L., Bross, I. D.: "Cigarette Smoking and Periodontal Disease," Journal American Dental Association, November, 1968, p. 1081.

PART I

DENTAL HEALTH EDUCATION AS INDIVIDUAL
LEARNING

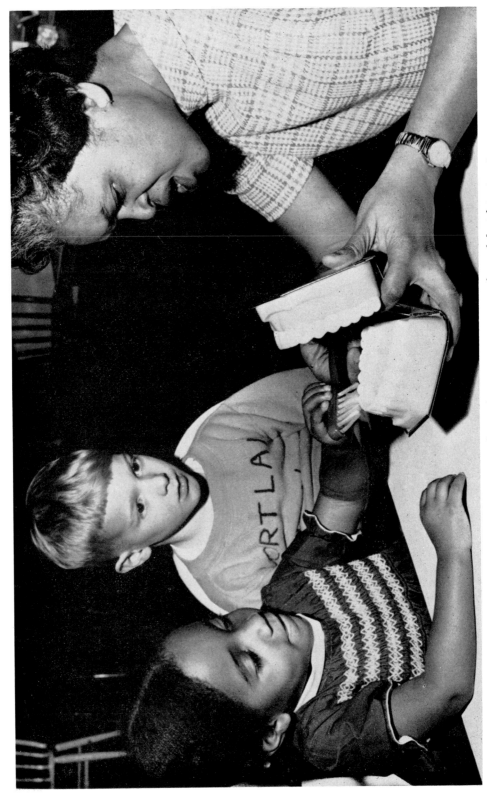

Fig. 3.—Underprivileged children need special attention to overcome fears of dental treatment.

Chapter 3

The Application of Psychological Concepts to Dental Health Instruction

Teeth are Troublesome

Teeth are a source of many disturbances, both physical and mental. Teeth represent pain and discomfort from the very beginning of life. The infant enjoys sucking but the breast-fed infant is deprived of this enjoyment as soon as he has teeth. He experiences pain in "cutting" teeth. He is disturbed emotionally when a primary tooth becomes loose and is exfoliated. The child may have deep fears about losing his primary teeth until mother reassures him that this is a natural process in growing up. Basically every one fears the loss of any member of the body including a tooth.

The mouth is a highly sensitive organ endowed with many sensory nerves. Emotions of affection, love, hate, cruelty and frustration may be associated with the mouth and teeth. This fact accounts for the change in attitude between the growing child and the young adult in accepting and then rejecting dental treatment. Frequently the eight- to ten-year olds accept dental treatment with little or no emotional concern, but there comes a time when he dislikes having his mouth and teeth manipulated. The adolescent is particularly sensitive about the mouth and teeth. He knows what he should do, but he dislikes having his teeth and mouth touched, so he rejects dental treatment until driven to the dentist by pain or other uncomfortable condition related to his mouth.

Child Development—The Changing Needs and Interests in Dental Health

Child development shows a constantly changing pattern of relationships in physical, mental and emotional growth. These changes vary from child to child, but it is possible to observe certain *patterns* of growth and development that are common to all children. Two factors should be kept in mind in dealing with children.

1. Accept the child as he is, but try to understand what he was like earlier in his life and how he may develop through proper guidance as he grows.

2. The child progresses from the home to the school and then to the community.

A characteristic of the preschool child is rapid growth of the body and the brain. He is learning to manage his bodily functions, such as elimination, saliva control and self-feeding, but he may be quite imperfect in performing these tasks. The child does not have complete eye-hand coordination or small muscle control, so it is pertinent to provide a toothbrush that is small and fits his hand, one that has a small brush head that he can safely and conveniently manipulate in his mouth. He should be taught to brush his teeth with large random strokes

15

because he lacks sufficient muscular control to learn more complicated ways of toothbrushing.

The preschool child is extremely active. He is beginning to develop memory, which signals his readiness to learn. He has a vivid imagination and is apt to be strongly self-assertive and self-centered. He likes to imitate, he accepts routine and enjoys repetition. These characteristics make him a good subject for learning dental health habits. Because he wants a measure of responsibility, he can be taught to brush his teeth directly after eating and to care for his toothbrush. He will enjoy a visit to the dentist if he is properly prepared before he is taken to the dental office and if the experience is a pleasant one.

Above all the preschool child must have a sense of security in his home and in the world into which he is venturing. He gains security by exploring new situations cautiously. Dental health instruction can add to a feeling of security as the child learns self-direction in acquiring daily dental health skills.

The child nine to eleven years old is absorbed in his own activities and those of his friends. He shows less interest in his parents, but he is still very dependent upon them for control and guidance. His interest in daily health routines is only mild and he needs frequent reminding to carry out good toothbrushing. The gang spirit is strong. He identifies with a specific group and wants no interference from adults in the group activities. The group sets his pattern of dress, speech and actions, but this is the time when indirect guidance from parents and teachers is sorely needed.

While this is a slower growth period than in the earlier years, it is a period of loss of primary teeth and the eruption and growth of the permanent teeth. The mouth may be uncomfortable during this period of growth although the child may not be consciously aware of the discomfort. He may rebel against brushing his teeth or any attempt to get him to the dentist. It is

also the period of high susceptibility to dental caries. Frequent trips to the dentist are necessary to control dental cavities that develop rapidly at this age. All possible preventive measures should be used to keep his mouth in a healthful condition.

What is an Adolescent?

Most people think of the adolescent as a teen-ager. Individual children may reach adolescence before the teen age, while others may not complete this growth period until they are almost twenty years of age. The Children's Bureau of the United States Department of Health, Education and Welfare defines adolescence as the period leading up to and for a number of years after a boy or girl has passed through changes that rise to a climax in sexual maturity. Because growing up is accomplished by young people in the years between the ages of twelve and twenty, it is convenient to call this period adolescence.

The signs of change in the life of the child are many. The adolescent's day is crammed with activity. He may show periods of furious activity and unpredictable spells of lackadaisical laziness. He seems at once a child and an adult, with constant shifting from one personality pattern to the other. Daydreaming, sudden periods of irritation, criticism of younger children in the family, discontent with all that is and wishing for all that is not characterizes this period of growth.

Adolescents have too much on their minds to think much about their health. It is difficult to motivate them to practice good health habits when most of them are enjoying good health. They do not eat a good diet as a rule. Considerable amounts of sugars and carbohydrates are consumed in an attempt to provide quick energy for the fast muscular activity and the emotional stress they experience.

Unless the adolescent has frequent, regular dental inspections and all the dental treatment necessary, he is subject to rampant dental decay and the onset of periodontal disease. All that was gained by good dental health habits and regular dental care during early childhood can be lost during the few years of neglect by the adolescent. Statistics show that by the time the average child reaches thirteen years of age, five permanent teeth have been attacked by dental caries. The number of permanent teeth affected continues to rise so that an average of seven teeth are affected by the time the adolescent is sixteen.

By intelligent guidance on the part of parents and teachers, good hygienic practices will carry over from childhood through adolescence and dental care will be accepted as part of growing up.

THE COMPONENTS OF ACTION

The Elements of Behavior

Behavior is defined as a series of choices among possible actions. Whether we examine the performance of a thoroughly familiar task such as toothbrushing or the individual's first attempts to solve a more complex problem such as accepting or rejecting dental treatment, the following elements are involved.

Situation. The situation presents alternatives requiring choice. The individual will tend to choose the situation that fulfills his need best.

Personal Characteristics. A person's abilities and attitudes limit the ways in which he can respond to situations, particularly when he is under stress, a factor which is present in most dental treatment.

Goal. The person sees some possibility of acting on the situation so as to gain satisfaction. Sometimes the aim is immediate gratification such as relief of pain. Other times it may be a delayed goal such as having a regular check-up and prophylaxis to ensure good dental health.

Interpretation. The person interprets a situation in accordance with the amount of knowledge he possesses about the subject under consideration. Before he acts, he must decide what actions are possible and what actions promise the best consequences.

Action. Few decisions to act are expected to result in complete satisfaction. Annoyances are expected to decrease the results of action, so the person must take whatever action will lead to the greatest satisfaction. For example, if the individual decides that going to the dentist and brushing his teeth regularly will make him more comfortable and socially acceptable, even though it takes time that he would rather spend in other activities, he will go to the dentist and faithfully brush his teeth. Conversely, if he does not see the values of good dental health, he will reject dental treatment and mouth hygiene.

Confirmation or Contradiction. The action is followed by the consequences which confirm or contradict the interpretation. If the person's experience in the dental office has been successful and satisfying and if the personalities of the dentist and other personnel in the office have been accepted by the patient, his decision to have dental treatment is confirmed. However, if the visit to the dentist has been unhappy or overly painful then the person's decision and action have been unsatisfactory. His decision, to his way of thinking, was a poor one. We say that his decision resulted in a contradiction, and he feels thwarted.

Reaction to Thwarting. When the person's actions fail to produce an adequately satisfying set of consequences, he is thwarted. He may try a new response; he may decide his goal cannot be reached. He may become emotionally upset. This reaction may be brought on by careless treatment or by thoughtless remarks during the dental visit. If the patient has been thwarted to the extent that he feels he cannot tolerate further treatment he will abandon further effort to obtain dental health and conclude that the goal cannot be reached. An interesting fact of behavior is illustrated in an article by Dr. Richard D. Sword. He says:

An immaculately groomed 47-year-old matron comes to the dental office for extensive dental treatment. She is cooperative and pleasant throughout her appointments. However, at the six-month recall examination it is found that she has neglected her mouth. Extensive calculus and soft debris are present. Recurrent decay is already evident at the margins of the gold restorations.

During the extensive treatment the patient has been advised about the importance of good oral hygiene that must be practiced on a regular routine. She has been shown the proper method of toothbrushing and other routines to maintain dental health. Why this neglect?

Because the two main factors of dental neglect, namely, poverty and ignorance, do not apply to this case, the answer must be in the emotional behavior of the individual. The author believes that it is a type of mental depression which manifests itself as "self-destruction" which in its less violent form becomes self-neglect. Because of unconscious guilt, a depressed patient may rationalize his behavior, that is, he may feel that he doesn't "deserve" dental treatment and oral health. When a patient repeatedly ignores advice and admonition concerning home care of teeth it may well be that a chronic depression is the underlying psychological process which prevents the individual from cooperating.[*]

Fear as a Deterrent to Dental Treatment

Any inquiry into the individual's attitudes should be for the purpose of increasing our ability to help him. In life there are three main fears, (1) fear of pain, (2) fear of loss of control and (3) fear of dismemberment and destruction.

People fear pain not only because of the physical discomfort but also because under the stress of pain the individual loses emotional control. Telling the person that part of his anatomy (a tooth) can decay and require extraction reminds him of the transient nature of life itself and the fear of dismemberment and destruction become very real. According to recent research

about 10 million Americans give fear as the primary reason for avoiding dental treatment and for failing to practice good dental hygiene. Such fears are not limited to any particular socioeconomic group. Fear accounts for many broken appointments.[†]

Expressive behavior, if it is carefully observed, will indicate the various ways in which the individual communicates his feeling of fear. He may squirm in the chair, constantly cross and uncross his legs, his hands may sweat or he may take extra firm hold on the arms of the chair.

Abnormal Behavior Patterns

The word psychosomatic is meant to imply a unity between "psycho," the mind, and "soma," the body. The psychosomatic theory of disease and health developed in medicine in the late 1930's as a reaction to the excessive biological emphasis that prevailed during the latter part of the nineteenth century, when great discoveries in bacteriology, pathology and biochemistry were made. A biological view of man prevailed. However, the human being, be he a medical or dental patient, is more than a collection of biological principles. The biological structure, the disease manifestations, the personality factors of the patient, the influence of his emotions, his presentation of himself and his response to treatment must be considered, not in bits and pieces but as a whole. Although great progress has been made in eliminating pain during dental treatment there still exists the problem of control of abnormal behavior caused by pain or fear of it.

In general, patients manifest seven types of psychosomatic tendencies.

1. *Anxiety.* As previously stated, fear is the dominant factor that influences the reaction of the anxious patient. It affects, to a greater or lesser degree, the behavior of the majority of those who seek dental treatment.

---

[*] Sword, R. O.: "Oral Neglect—Why?" Journal American Dental Association, June, 1970, p. 1327.

[†] Gale, E. N., Ayer, W. A.: "Treatment of Dental Phobias," Journal American Dental Association, June, 1969, p. 1304.

2. *Chronic Complaints.* This behavior is frequently seen among persons who wear dentures. The reaction is probably due to the residue of fear of the loss of bodily members—the teeth. After hearing the complaint and making all necessary adjustments, the dentist should be sympathetically firm to help the patient accept the substitute for his natural teeth.

3. *Hysteria.* This behavior is characteristic of females and is a learned response to any disturbing situation. A firm but sympathetic attitude usually helps to quiet the patient. It is very difficult to get these patients to relax so that work is usually accomplished under conditions of stress. Appointments should be short. The frequency and length of visits may be increased after the patient shows favorable response to treatment and after the hysteria becomes less frequent. Premedication helps in extreme cases.

4. *Obsession.* This behavior is manifested by the patient who tries to cover insecurity and fear with a "know-it-all" attitude. He reacts the same in all situations in which he does not excel. He demands a full explanation of everything that is to be done, questioning every detail of treatment. He is apt to be a person who has tried many dental offices and has been unwelcome in some of them. After a complete explanation of the treatment planned, he must be told to accept or reject the plan offered. Usually he will accept, but the pattern of insecure behavior will persist.

5. *Paranoia.* This behavior is manifested by patients who have undue, extreme suspicion of everything and everyone. He is sure that something has gone wrong during treatment and is in constant need of reassurance. A calm attitude of assurance on the part of the dentist and staff helps to allay the suspicions which this individual has difficulty in controlling.

6. *Meticulous Brushing.* This behavior is shown by the individual who overcleans his mouth. Many times, such a person keeps his teeth meticulously clean, but has no thought or interest in having them repaired. Removing the "dirt" from the teeth seems to satisfy the urge to rid the body of unclean thoughts or actions. The person is using toothbrushing as a way of ridding the mind of guilt feelings.

7. *Self-pity.* For the person who displays this behavior, the teeth are frequently the focus of self-pity. His attitude says "I don't suppose there is much I can do about my teeth. I inherited soft teeth from my mother." What the person is really trying to say is, in effect, "Look at me, I am suffering so much because I have bad teeth." This pattern can also be seen in other incidents in the person's life. It is a pattern developed to overcome insecurity or to excuse it. Patience, kindness and firmness helps but will not cure the person of this behavior pattern.

Psychology of Motivation

There are a great many internal as well as external forces that affect what a person does, how he feels and how he thinks. These are called *needs*. They range from basic drives such as hunger, thirst, sex and freedom from discomfort to needs which originate in social situations such as acceptance, recognition, leadership and companionship. The fulfillment of these motivating forces serves to satisfy the need and to relieve tension. Psychologists agree that all the patterns of behavior are motivated. In some instances the motives are easily identified; in others, it is difficult to understand the hidden motives that prompt persons to behave as they do.

The process of motivation has four major factors:

1. the need or drive
2. action by the individual
3. a goal or incentive to be achieved
4. some form of satisfaction

If any step in the process is missing, the process will stop and frustration will take the place of motivation. For example, a notice for a six-month prophylaxis and checkup is sent to a patient. He knows he should have his teeth cleaned at this time (the need). He calls for an appointment and arrives at the office on time (action). He has his teeth cleaned and x-rayed (goal achieved). He has the pleasant feeling of a clean mouth and having done what was necessary to have a healthy mouth (satisfaction).

If he fails to get an appointment within a reasonable length of time or if he himself fails to keep the appointment, there is a break in the motivational force. It is necessary to start over again, either by a second reminder or by his phoning for another appointment—if he has not lost the initial motivation in the meantime.

There are a great many sources of motivation. Some of these are *physiological* and originate in the body. They are directed toward keeping the body at an optimal degree of health and efficiency, maintaining body balance so that all systems are "go". In some individuals the basic physiological drives are linked to good mouth hygiene while in others such motivation is lacking. They do not seek dental health until driven to it by pain.

Motives may be modified by social pressures or by personal preference. These are *learned* motivations. The person wants social acceptance so he keeps his teeth clean and in good repair. Or, he may go a step further and practice good dental hygiene, working for the secondary goal of maintaining healthy teeth to avoid the more basic problem of avoiding pain.

Society places many restrictions upon the individual. Some of these such as brushing the teeth to prevent mouth odors are customs which society demands for social acceptance. Others are mores built into a certain society. The amount of dental literature produced to motivate people to take care of their teeth or suffer the dire consequences to health and social prestige is a strong force in shaping the mores of our culture.

Some individuals practice good mouth hygiene to fulfill the desire for *recognition*. This may be a force among adolescents who dress, act and react as the group demands. If good dental health makes a boy or girl more acceptable, then you may be sure it will be practiced diligently.

Desire for dependency. This is seen in individuals who make more than the required visits to the physician or dentist just to be sure everything is all right. This is a form of dependency from which a person derives some measure of satisfaction and security. The desire for attention is strong and he is willing to pay for it.

Negative motivators are seen in the form of fear. The person accepts dental treatment, although he does not want it, because of the fear of tooth loss and the prospect of wearing dentures.

Factors in Interpersonal Relationships

It is necessary to understand that relationships are based on individual needs, motivation and behavior patterns. When we observe specific reactions by one person we are receiving "cues" that help us to understand him. We come to know the people around us more intimately through these cues. We all learn very early the meaning of a frown and the significance of a smile. Such cues have a bearing on the motivational state of the individual or give insight into hidden or subconscious needs and motives. They may not be evident to the individual manifesting the behavior.

The ability to observe behavioral cues and relate them to an understanding of specific modes of behavior is a great asset in instructing and treating patients. Rudeness by a patient may be a manifestation of an intense feeling of anxiety. He may be unable to deal successfully with this emotion and he reacts with undesirable behavior. If we are aware of the person as an individual with feelings that he displays as nonverbal cues, we can act accordingly and relieve tension.

Interpersonal relations are improved by a positive approach. The ability to relate to others with warmth and understanding increases our confidence in treating their dental problems successfully. A positive response requires a friendly attitude, a warm personal approach and a feeling of empathy for the patient's immediate needs. Calling the person by his name is a very important part of a positive approach. It indicates concern and understanding.

The Power of Persuasion

There are many approaches to good personal relations. The one that applies best to dental health education is *persuasion*. The first step is to be a good listener. Give the patient time to talk about himself and his problems. Let him express opinions that may lead to revealing prejudices and preconceived notions regarding dental health and treatment. Then the patient can be instructed in a manner which will not tear down his opinions but will offer better ideas which he can accept voluntarily. Criticism has no value in this situation. The goal of persuasion is to change the behavior of the individual by having him accept a concept of dental health which heretofore was unfamiliar to him. Attitudes are difficult to change but with the proper "gentle persuasion" a great deal can be accomplished. For example, a patient needs to brush his teeth more thoroughly and at regular times during the day. Just telling him so will not bring results and may injure his self-esteem. By offering evidence in the form of some type of visual experience, such as the use of disclosing wafers to show the plaque and debris remaining on the teeth, he can be convinced that he is not doing the job expected of him. A thought or idea has been offered. The next step is to create the desire for a clean mouth. A thorough prophylaxis will give the patient the pleasant experience of having a clean mouth. Acceptance of the idea of more regular cleaning follows. The result will be that the patient wants to brush his teeth because he is convinced he has something to gain by doing so. The result has been accomplished *indirectly* by motivating him to desire a clean mouth.

Understanding the Underprivileged

Our present society is in a state of turmoil. We are being apprised of the need to understand our minority groups, the underprivileged, and the uneducated. Basically their needs are the same as those of other members of the population. They lack the means of meeting these needs. Society is challenged to reach these groups with effective education so that they will seek self-realization through their own efforts. They must be assisted through mutual understanding.

Dr. Clifton Dummett says: "Because the success and efficacy of health care are dependent on the cooperation of those who need care, there must be more mutual understanding between consumer (the patient) and the provider (the dentist). Understanding that many diverse conditions and persons exist in disadvantaged areas is an important step in closing the communication gap. Furthermore, the poor should be consulted and must be involved in planning and carrying out health programs that affect them specifically."[*]

The reactions of the disadvantaged people to many situations are different from the responses of more fortunate members of our society. They agree among themselves in regard to attitudes, superstitions and values concerning their own health and the health of their neighbors. Some of the negative attitudes of the poor have been identified as:

1. hypersensitive attitudes during clinical treatment;
2. over-reaction to imagined grievances;
3. testing of persons whose motives are not clear;
4. resentment and reactions to certain physical contacts;

[*] Dummett, C. O.: "Understanding the Underprivileged Patient," Journal American Dental Association, December, 1969, p. 1363.

5. communication gaps;
6. fears about dental treatment;
7. confusion concerning health concepts.[*]

Through experience it has been learned that the poor seek health services, including dental care, only as a last resort, after all other means have failed. Fatalism is common among this group. It requires a great deal of effort to convince them that teeth are worth saving.

Unless professionals agree to involve the underprivileged in the planning of health programs there will continue to be large communication gaps. The poor often have very intelligent opinions and suggestions concerning health planning that fit their needs. If they are included as members of the health team, a long step forward will be made in recognizing their needs and fulfilling them.

Conclusion

It would take a great deal more space than this text allows to cover the important subject of the psychological implications of patient management. An attempt has been made to give an overview of the problems and some possible solutions that may be effective in understanding the needs and motivations of those treated and instructed in clinics and dental offices. Keeping in mind that each person is a unique individual who requires special study and understanding is of paramount importance.

Present-day practice in professional education tends to overlook the psychological approach to patient management because courses in the science of human behavior are taught as *preparatory to* rather than *in conjunction with* the clinical application of dental science. It is hoped that the ideas in this chapter will be used by clinical instructors to prepare students for clinical service and to provide a background for

[*] Trithart, C. O.: "Understanding the Underprivileged Child," Report of an Experimental Workshop, Journal American Dental Association, October, 1968, p. 880.

further clinical observations and studies by students.

Questions for Review and Discussion

1. Explain the relationship of teeth to individual sensitivity (a) in early childhood (b) in adults.

2. Name the factors that guide the initial relationship with a child.

3. State briefly the characteristics of (a) a child four or five years old, (b) a child nine to eleven years old, (c) an adolescent.

4. How would you prepare a child three years old for his first visit to the dental office? What circumstances should be avoided?

5. Describe a patient who exhibits *normal behavior patterns* while receiving dental treatment (thought question).

6. Define behavior.

7. Name the components which lead to action.

8. What causes the reaction known as "thwarting"?

9. Discuss Sword's interpretation of oral neglect in terms of psychological manifestations. Recall instances in your own experience that might collaborate this theory.

10. Name some of the observable mannerisms that indicate personal fear during dental treatment.

11. Name the four factors inherent in the process of motivation.

12. Discuss what is meant by "cues" in interpersonal relations.

13. What is empathy?

14. Write a short paper using the technique of persuasion to convince a fearful person that dental treatment is a necessary part of obtaining good dental health.

15. Discuss dental prophylaxis as a means of relating positively to the individual.

16. There are seven attitudes unique to the underprivileged. Appoint seven members of the class to discuss each of these and give suggestions for changing or avoiding such attitudes.

Selected Readings

Blum, L. H.: "Doctor-Patient Relationship in Psychological Perspective of Transference-Counter Transference," Part I, New York Journal of Dentistry, April, 1970, p. 125, Part II May, 1970, p. 167.

Cinotti, W. R., Grieder, A.: APPLIED PSYCHOLOGY IN DENTISTRY, C. V. Mosby Co., St. Louis, 1964, Chapters 7, 12.

Colt, A. M.: "Elements of Comprehensive Health Planning," American Journal of Public Health, July, 1970, p. 1194.

Finn, Sidney B.: CLINICAL PEDODONTICS, W. B. Saunders Co., Philadelphia, 1967, Chapter 2, p. 19.

Gale, E. N., Ayer, W. A.: "Treatment of Dental Phobias," Journal American Dental Association, June, 1969, p. 1304.

Heyns, R. W.: THE PSYCHOLOGY OF PERSONAL ADJUSTMENT, Holt, Rinehart & Winston, New York, 1958, Chapter 12.

Kiesler, C. A., Nesbitt, R. E., Zanna, M. P.: "On Inferring One's Beliefs for One's Behavior," Journal of Personality and Social Pyschology, November, 1969, p. 231.

Raynor, J. F.: "Socioeconomic Status and Factors Influencing the Dental Health Practices of Mothers," American Journal of Public Health, July, 1970, p. 1250.

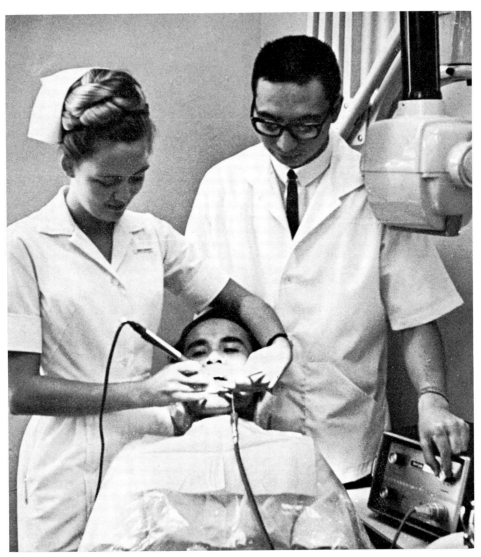

FIG. 4.—The team approach to dental health involves all members of the dental office staff in the education of the patient. (Courtesy, Department of Dental Hygiene, University of Hawaii.)

Chapter 4

Opportunities for Individual Instruction During Dental Treatment

The Educative Moment

The education of the patient begins with the telephone call for the first appointment and continues at a steady, measured rate through every appointment. Opportunities for educating the patient are endless because the science of dental health is continually growing, with new processes for treatment, new methods of prevention and new concepts of mouth hygiene.

The dental office or clinic provides an *educative moment* when the patient is in a highly receptive state of mind to accept or reject dental treatment. He wants to know and he wants to know now! What is to be done in his mouth? How will it affect his general health? What may he expect in the future? These are but a few of the thoughts that go through the patient's mind in his attempt to arrive at the right decisions.

The instruction efforts in the dental office have several aims. They are:

1. to place the patient in a relaxed, receptive state of mind so that he will accept dental treatment in an atmosphere of confidence.

2. to impart scientific information in lay language so that he will understand the meaning of dental service and place the proper value upon it in terms of continuing optimal dental health,

3. to make an effort to motivate the patient to practice good dental health habits,

4. to correct unfavorable attitudes that may exist from previous dental experiences, misinformation and superstitions.

The Team Approach to Teaching Dental Health

The dentist has full authority over what should be taught; how it should be taught and who shall do the teaching. He must decide the philosophy of the office as to the time allowed for instruction; the items he wishes to be included in each visit; he must, in general, "set the curriculum" for all who are to teach. There are two philosophies concerning patient instruction that prevail in dental offices.

Plan 1. All the instruction is given by the dentist. He feels that this is such an important area of service that it can not be delegated to other personnel. The dentist spends two or more appointments, one-half hour each, conditioning the patient for good dental health procedures to be carried out at home and for diagnosis and discussion of the complete treatment plan and follow-up procedures. For this service the patient is charged a fee. After the dentist has completed the restorative work, the follow-up and the dental health procedures, prophylaxis and X rays with further instruction are delegated to the dental hygienist and the assistant under supervision of the dentist.

Plan 2. During the first visit, the dentist meets the patient for an examination and a get-acquainted discussion. The patient is given prophylaxis and X rays are taken by the dental hygienist. Discussion of the home care routine completes the first visit. Return visits are concerned with complete diagnosis, treatment planning and discussion of fees. The patient pays for the prophylaxis and the X rays. In this plan the auxiliaries do most of the instruction. The dentist's limited time is considered more valuable for providing restorative care for a greater number of patients. In either case emergencies are treated immediately to alleviate pain.

The Environment of the Dental Suite

The general physical environment of the dental suite produces lasting impressions upon the new patient. Ideally, an attractive waiting room, like an attractive home, should have a feeling of quiet comfort—not ominous silence! Walls should be in a pleasant color that blends with the furnishings. Good pictures should complement the walls. Furniture should be comfortable and easy to maintain and clean. Adequate, restful lighting helps a great deal in making the patient comfortable. Current dental literature written for lay people should be available on a take-it-as-you-leave basis. The short time, and it should be only a few minutes, that the patient is seated in the waiting room is an excellent opportunity for motivating him toward better dental health practices. This should not be wasted on back issues of magazines. By all means keep dental literature current, with recent issues available for return patients. Even dental and other professional health journals will be read by the more informed persons. Dental health literature should not have to compete with popular magazines for attention. They should be placed on separate tables or stands, with dental health materials given the more conspicuous place. The philosophy of the dental practice is frequently revealed to the patient by what he reads in the reception room. Most patients appreciate the opportunity to learn since they cannot always ask intelligent questions on subjects that puzzle them. A few brief statements gleaned from a pam-

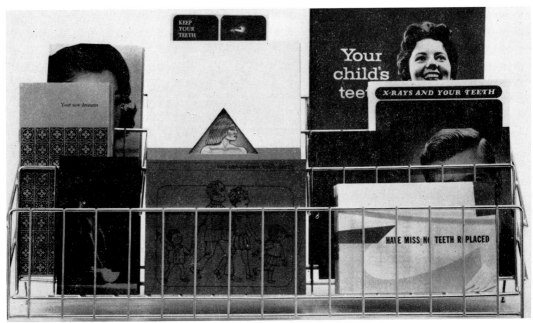

Fig. 5.—Attractively arranged dental health literature provided in the waiting room. (Copyright by the American Dental Association, Reprinted by permission.)

phlet, magazine or picture are a valuable contribution to the patient's education.

Topics on home care, preventive measures, community problems of dental health, dental care for children, the value of periodic checkups and nutrition information are but a few of the subjects of general interest. Convincing articles on community water fluoridation may reach skeptical persons. Short articles on newer methods of treatment written for lay people tend to give confidence in the treatment received. If the patient reads about it in the dental office, it follows that the dentist knows about the new methods and probably uses them. Americans read a lot and the influence of the written word should be used to the fullest advantage in the dental office.

The entire dental suite should be free of unpleasant distractions such as traffic noises, inadequate ventilation and uncomfortable temperature. Odors that infiltrate from the dental laboratory and the operating rooms into the waiting room may be quite distressing to the waiting patient. No longer does the dental suite represent the sterile, cold, unfriendly atmosphere of a hospital. New operatories conceal all equipment, provide comfortably balanced dental chairs and a number of pain- and fear-reducing devices. All are intended to give the patient a sense of security.

The Dentist as an Educator

The dentist's chairside personality is usually formed and somewhat crystallized by the time he leaves dental school. It is not separate and distinct from his own personality, but a chairside manner can be cultivated. What do people expect in a dentist? First and foremost they seek an individual who has excellent technique; one who has a good reputation in his community and among his professional colleagues. Personality traits are a secondary consideration. The successful dentist has a fine balance between good professional attitude and friendliness. He should be willing to explain what he is doing in the patient's mouth as he works. How can a person appreciate what is done for him if he does not know what is being done? If the patient is to have appreciation for dental service he must know what he needs; why he needs it; and he must be given some idea of the difficulties incident to providing the treatment. An appreciative patient is an informed one.

The Dental Hygienist as an Educator

The dental profession recognizes the dental hygienist as the professional aide, qualified by education and state examinations to perform health services for the patient. The primary function of the dental hygienist is to interpret dental health facts and procedures in lay language so that the patient will be conditioned to practice good dental health habits. She establishes good rapport with the patient, giving him confidence in her services and those of the dentist. In many offices the dental prophylaxis, the scaling and polishing of teeth, is the first treatment received by the patient. Most dentists require patients to have a clean mouth before treatment is started. The patient gains a good impression of the working relationships in the dental office and the attitudes of dental personnel toward him as an individual. He learns what is expected of him in the total care of his own mouth.

In preparing the patient for further dental treatment, the dental hygienist may take a comprehensive case history and in some cases may obtain facts pertinent to treatment that may have escaped the dentist. Patients will frequently confide in the dental hygienist information withheld during dental interviews. She understands the significance of total health in relation to dental health and may bring to the dentist's attention conditions she finds during the prophylaxis. She teaches with scientific accuracy not only dental health facts and procedures but assesses individual nutritional needs and diet control. She may recommend preventive measures such as topical applications of medicaments for the prevention of dental decay. As one who renders treatment and instruction, the dental hygienist is a valuable member of the dental health team.

The Education of the Patient by Other Members of the Dental Team

Patients meet a variety of people: the clerks in clinics; the dental assistants, secretaries, and office managers in private practice. They contribute to dental health education in a number of different ways. The information they provide should be authentic and in agreement with the professional opinions of the dentist and the dental hygienist. They are not responsible for patient instruction but they must give clear, concise directions and information based on the philosophy of the particular office. Clinics and dental offices depend on them for smooth handling of patients, effective use of time and a general atmosphere of cooperation and efficiency.

Unless the auxiliary personnel have adequate education in dental health instruction methods and procedures, they should not attempt to discuss dental treatment, dental pathology, mouth hygiene or diet control with the patient. If they take X rays they should be well informed in the science of roentgenology.

The dentist who permits the auxiliary personnel to instruct the patient in toothbrushing and home care techniques is relegating the most important part of dental health to a less than important status in the mind of the patient. Only the dentist and dental hygienist are qualified to teach these important routines and to check at each recall appointment how effectively the patient has performed the home care of his mouth and teeth.

The areas in which auxiliary personnel are particularly knowledgeable are as follows: making appointments; providing written instructions for postoperative home care; discussing the payment of fees, and the recall procedures. These functions con-

tribute to the information that the patient receives and they are vital to the smooth, efficient operation of the office or clinic.

The Telephone in Patient Education

The telephone call for an appointment is the first contact a new patient has with the dental office of his choice. It is an opportunity to establish good relations with a new patient. He needs to feel assured that he is welcome. When he hears a pleasant voice he knows that the dental personnel have a feeling of sincerity and interest in him as an individual.

When arranging an appointment for a new patient it is important to obtain his full name, address, home and business telephone numbers, the name of the person who referred him and what his immediate problem is. A short appointment at the earliest possible time will usually take care of an emergency. If the person requests complete dental services on a continuing basis, a full-length appointment should be made to allow for consultation with the dentist, X rays, prophylaxis, and possibly, study models. If this is the office routine it should be explained to the patient.

The First Appointment

A new patient's first appointment will in most cases determine whether he will return for future treatment. It is essential that the dentist see the person as soon as possible after he arrives at the office. A friendly professional approach by everyone will impress the patient favorably toward continuing his appointments.

Sufficient time should be allowed to discuss the patient's dental problems. The patient should be informed concerning the routine followed in the office. If he is to be charged for a broken appointment, explain that it means lost time and income for the dentist. The patient then will be more likely to keep his appointments or cancel them far enough in advance so that the time may be reassigned. When a patient comes to the office for the first time he expects to have something done. As mentioned above, X rays, prophylaxis and study models provide a good approach to future patient relationship. It also gives the new patient time to make decisions as to future dental treatment.

Instruction During Prophylactic Treatment by a Dental Hygienist

Prevention of many dental diseases can be accomplished by a good routine of mouth hygiene. The dental prophylaxis is a prerequisite for a clean mouth and provides an opportunity for extensive patient instruction. Sufficient time for this should be allowed not only at the first treatment but also during all recall treatments.

The dental hygienist is a trained educator. She has a unique advantage for instructing the patient during a treatment that should be pleasant and refreshing. The feeling of a clean mouth is a good motivating force for further effort on the part of the patient in accepting his role in performing good dental health habits. The dental hygienist should use as many visual aids as possible, including one of normal dentition so that a comparison can be made with his own teeth and gingival conditions. The patient must know *why* it is important to brush the teeth, *when* to brush and *how* to manipulate the toothbrush so as to completely remove food debris, dental plaque and to stimulate the gingiva. The patient may be introduced to other means of mouth cleaning such as the dental tape, interdental stimulators, water sprays and disclosing tablets. Practice sessions are advised whenever a patient is to begin using one of these instruments. It should not be assumed that he knows how to use it.

The patient's diet should be discussed as an individual problem. It is an important aspect of dental health instruction. It is good to have some idea of the patient's food habits so that the dentist may give specific instruction to the dental hygienist regarding possible changes in diet. If the restriction of free sugars is indicated or if tests for caries susceptibility are indicated, the hygienist may make such tests and give nutritional advice.

The dental hygienist should show interest in the patient's questions, answer them intelligently but briefly. Overtalking tires most people. It takes many appointments to cover all the areas of instruction that a patient needs. At the end of the first complete prophylaxis, which may take more than one appointment, recall schedules should be discussed with the idea of finding times which are most convenient for the patient. The desired outcome is an appreciative patient who understands the value of good home routine for dental health and who returns for periodic dental prophylaxis, oral examination and any dental treatment that may be necessary.

Instruction During the X-ray Survey

Every one has been alerted to the threat of environmental contamination. The effect of radiation on the human body has been dramatized to a point where some dental patients have refused to have dental X rays. It is important to allay fears and to correct erroneous ideas concerning the annual x-ray survey and the bite-wing films taken at each recall appointment. The United States Public Health Service will inspect dental office equipment upon request to determine the amount of radiation to which the patient and the operator are exposed. Where equipment is found unsafe by emitting rays that are harmful, corrections should be made. Aluminum filters for the older type of machines are usually the only correction needed. New equipment has all the safeguards built in. In some cases the room in which the machine is installed may require corrections. If these precautions have been taken the patient should be told to set his mind at ease. Lead aprons for patient protection are considered desirable, particularly when the patients are pregnant.

The x-ray machine is an interesting part of dental equipment. It should be used to educate the patient. Explain the short time of exposure required with the fast films. Show the patient the film pack *before* placing it in his mouth. Explain the exposure of films. Use a hand mirror to show the patient the conditions in his mouth that require X rays so that he will understand why they are taken. Explain the advantage of X rays in making a precise diagnosis and explain that additional films may be needed as dental treatment progresses.

Before placing the film in the patient's mouth, take time to instruct him how to control his breath, throat and mouth muscles, and how to relax his jaws and tongue. Show him how to avoid gagging. While the films are being exposed, keep him interested in what is being done so that he will not mind the immediate discomfort.

Patients like to see their films, even though they may not understand them. It is a good idea to have a set of films showing nearly perfect teeth so that comparisons can be made with the patient's own films. The results of careful instruction concerning dental X rays will tend to reduce a patient's resistance because of the cost and he will expect the service at stated intervals.

Operative Dental Procedures—A Time for Learning

Dental treatment is a mystery to most patients. Some patients want to know exactly what is going on; others prefer not to know what is being done. In order to place the patient at ease it is necessary to know what type of person he is and to instruct him accordingly. Sometimes, despite all efforts to make the environment tension-free, the fear of pain and of the unknown may still persist.

The patient who is to have a cavity prepared for filling should be told beforehand that all precautions against causing pain will be used. He should be prepared for the injection of local anesthetic. The dentist should explain why it is used, how it is administered, and how the patient must react before the anesthetic wears off.

The patient will appreciate hearing about the high-speed equipment and the fast-cutting burs while the cavity preparation continues. The patient knows what the dentist is doing so that he forgets about his anxiety. When the filling material is prepared it is good to explain why a certain filling is best for the particular cavity. Frequently a saliva ejector is placed in the patient's mouth without instruction as to how to control it during treatment. A saliva ejector can be very uncomfortable, especially in the mouths of young children and old patients, unless they are shown how to control it. When cotton rolls and rubber dams are used, the dentist should explain that they keep the area clean and dry and that the patient must be quiet so that the dentist can work quickly. If impressions are to be taken, the dentist should explain the process and how the patient can assist by controlling his breathing.

There are many areas of operative treatment that offer opportunities for patient instruction, but there is one time in the course of the dentist-patient relationship that is particularly dependent on a good presentation—oral diagnosis and treatment planning. Unless the patient is given complete information at this time, he will very likely reconsider whether the treatment suggested is worth the effort in time, money and future benefits. The patient frequently asks questions of other members of the office staff which he is embarrassed to ask of the dentist. The auxiliaries should know the answers to those questions which are not highly technical, such as how long the whole treatment will take, how much time each appointment requires and many questions about payment of fees. They are all important to the patient and should receive considerate answers. The more technical questions should be referred to the dentist.

Instruction for the Surgical Patient

Extraction of a tooth is a major surgical operation and should be treated as such. No one undergoes surgery without fear.

Psychologically, the patient is faced with the loss of a part of his body, a frightening prospect! During the operation, the dentist should keep all instruments out of the patient's view. He should calm the patient with a quiet voice. Move rapidly and silently. Talk as little as possible. Feel confidence in yourself and the patient will sense your ability to care for him. A cooperative patient is a help to the surgeon. There are less emotional after-effects and recovery is hastened. A calm mind improves healing and lessens postoperative discomfort.

All instructions for preoperative and postoperative conduct should be written in simple, positive and clear language. After the operation impress the patient with his responsibility in the healing process. Give him exact information for reaching the surgeon in case of postoperative emergencies. The fees may seem very high for the time that the operation takes. Explain to the patient that he is paying for the surgeon's skill and judgement, not merely for the time involved.

The Denture Patient is Special

Patients who are being fitted with new dentures have progressed through a series of dental experiences which include restoration of any teeth that can be saved and surgical procedures for removal of teeth, bone and soft tissues. Many of these patients are in the older age group and many may be suffering from emotional disturbances due to age. Their tissues have lost the tone and elasticity of youth. They are slow to recover and slower still to accept change. These conditions make it difficult to treat the geriatric patient. Most of them have been through an emotional crisis at the thought of losing most or all of their teeth. It is necessary to show particular concern for the improvement of the mental attitude of the denture patient. Artificial appliances never function as well as natural teeth. They are at best 75% efficient. The dentist should explain that

dentures are not permanent "fixtures." They need frequent adjustment and occasional replacement. Facial contours change in the aging process, but dentures are not usually the cause of such changes. Better methods of construction and a variety of tooth forms make dentures resemble the natural teeth more closely. Dentures can be *individualized* so that they are not easily detected.

A small room or alcove, with soft lighting and a sitting room atmosphere, is often used for the first fitting of a new denture. This setting tends to cushion the shock and places the patient in a comfortable living atmosphere where he will be seen with the denture. "Before" and "after" photographs may help to convince the denture patient that there has been a marked improvement in his appearance.

Take time to instruct the patient in how to speak with the new appliance and how to care for the denture at home to prevent stains and denture odors. Do not assume that he knows about the care of a denture. Give explicit directions including the type of cleanser to be used, when to use it and how to use it. Most patients have difficulty in eating at first. The dental team should have full knowledge of suitable diets and how to control mastication. Written instructions are good since there is much to remember and the older patient does not have a long memory span. When the patient comes in for adjustments encourage him to talk about his difficulties. In younger patients fear of detection is often a more serious consideration than the fit of the appliance. Patience and encouragement go a long way in dispelling worry and fear.

The denture patient who has been properly conditioned by education during the many steps that go into making a denture should come to the end of the experience better prepared for speaking, eating and he should be in better health. The dentist should give service willingly until the patient is completely satisfied with the results.

A satisfied denture patient is a good recommendation for a dental practice.

Child Management in Dental Practice

There are two specialties in dental practice that deal with children. Pedodontics, the treatment of children from infancy to adolescence, and orthodontics, the treatment of malformations and malplacement of teeth. Many children are treated by specialists. However, the majority of children are treated by general practitioners. It is not the intent of this text to discuss in depth the subject of child management, but rather to give some general observations on the management of the child as patient in general practice.

When a child is placed in an unfamiliar environment he resorts to the natural urge, self-preservation. The first emotion in an unknown situation is fear. A child experiences several kinds of fear when he is faced with the possibility of having a stranger handle him; the reaction is to resist. Fear of the unknown; fear of pain; fear of ridicule call forth the urge to flee from the situation. Control of fear must be undertaken before the child comes to the dental office. The parent should assure the child that he will be safe in this new experience.

Once the child is assured and convinced that the experience will be pleasant he becomes an interested patient and the dental visit no longer calls forth fear reactions. It is most important that nothing in the handling of the child disturbs the confidence built up by an understanding parent. The child that is seen in most dental offices has had some introduction to dental health concepts in his home and perhaps in school. He knows that teeth need attention. He hears about other children's experiences (not always pleasant). When he finds himself in an adult situation, he hopes to act like an adult. Treating children with the same respect as an adult is a sound philosophy of child management. A child respects those who respect him. He likes to be spoken to as though

he understood what is going on, even if he doesn't quite understand. He wants to be treated in a way that he will have a satisfactory personal experience.

Dental services for children are expensive in time and energy and must be paid for on that basis. Whenever a child visits a dental office he should have some treatment. As his confidence increases, so also will the amount of treatment accomplished. He learns to accept slight physical discomfort for the satisfaction of parental approval and other immediate tangible rewards. The question of reward for good behavior has been challenged. Good behavior is expected and therefore should not be purchased with a reward. However, a child may be given a small gift at the end of the first visit to show that the dentist is his friend. A box of small toys is offered and the child may make his own selection. This procedure also prevents the tendency of younger children to want some of the larger and more valuable books, games and toys from the children's corner in the waiting room.

The Children's Corner

The child's initial contact with the dental office is in the reception room. In order to make the child feel at home it has been the practice in some offices to provide a special corner or section in the reception room equipped for children. Small chairs, tables, books, pictures, and "handling" objects such as dolls, small toys and puzzles give the child something to do and a feeling of belonging. In addition some dental materials that will be used such as cotton rolls, saliva ejector, paper cups, rubber polishing cups, a mouth mirror and x-ray film may be placed on the table. Becoming acquainted with these articles before he enters the operatory is helpful. A book for children which shows only one instrument which will be used during treatment on a page, with just a few words about it, will help the parent to keep the child's interest while he is waiting. A small coat hanger and a hook in the coat closet placed so that he can hang up his own coat is another way to make him feel that he belongs in this new place.

Dental Prophylaxis—A Learning Experience for Children

Having teeth cleaned at the first dental appointment is a pleasant way of introducing a child to dental treatment. He learns about dental equipment firsthand and feels the pleasant sensation of a clean mouth. He learns to accept the manipulation of his mouth and teeth. The child is properly conditioned for his first appointment with the dentist. The dental cleaning also serves to motivate him to brush his teeth routinely at home, for he is told that his teeth will be checked for good brushing at the next appointment. Using a disclosing solution or tablets with a hand mirror the dentist or the dental hygienist can show the child the stains and how they are removed.

Educational Outcomes of Dental Health Instruction

As constant learning goes on in the dental office, a child may be expected to learn some basic concepts that should remain with him throughout life. Some of these are:

1. The dentist is his friend, and he is considerate and understanding.

2. Cooperation and good behavior shorten the dental visit.

3. He is responsible for the health of his teeth through regular, careful toothbrushing.

4. Avoiding accidents to his teeth is important.

5. Good food is necessary for good health so he should accept the food provided at meal time.

6. An excessive amount of sugar, especially between meals, is the main cause of tooth decay.

7. Acceptance of dental treatment on a regular basis and willingness to give up some of his spare time for the benefits of good dental health is part of growing up.

8. He needs to know about teeth and their importance to good general health.

Suggestions Concerning Dental Treatment for Children

Most children will accept dental treatment if the following guidelines are followed:

1. Appointments for young children are scheduled in the early morning when they are rested and quiet. The dentist is better able to cope with the children's problems at this time of day.

2. Older children are given early afternoon appointments so that their playtime is not forfeited for dental treatment.

3. Short appointments are necessary if a child has a short interest span. Appointments may be lengthened as he matures.

4. Give the nervous child longer intervals between visits so that he may not be subjected to periods of nervous tension too often.

5. Be truthful to children about dental pain. Respect their tolerance. Work quickly but avoid the tension that builds up if the work is hurried.

6. Use every available means to reduce discomfort.

7. Do not play with a child in the dental situation. He is in a serious mood and wants to be treated accordingly.

Special Problems of Adolescents

The teen-ager is frequently as difficult to treat as the young child, particularly if he has not had regular dental treatment during his early years. He may be over-talkative or completely silent. In either case he is trying to control fear. Yet he does not acknowledge fear to himself and he wants no one to suspect that he is afraid. Both boys and girls are highly emotional during puberty and their tolerance of pain is low. They have a longer period of endurance than the younger children, but they may suffer a degree of shock due to tension if put to the test. In treating adolescents, keep as much equipment out of sight as possible. They are highly susceptible to impressions. Emotional tension causes fainting in the teen-ager.

Boys and girls of this age are seeking career information. Some are interested in science, others in technology. They will enjoy watching the work that goes on in a dental laboratory. The x-ray equipment can be a most rewarding experience if it is properly presented as a form of scientific advancement in dentistry. This is an excellent opportunity to interest them in dental careers. The time spent in educating the adolescent will serve to build an appreciation for the art and science, and the values and costs, of dentistry. A great deal of talk goes on among teen-agers. They will listen to explanations for hours on end. Use the time you are working in the mouth to explain procedures; to impart dental health facts and to increase their interest in the long-term goals of dental health.

CAUTION! Drug Addiction

In this day of experimentation among teen-agers, particularly with drugs, dental personnel have an excellent opportunity to observe and teach prevention and recognition of the use of drugs. Every one should know the physical and emotional signs of drug addiction. Recognizing and reporting to the dentist deviations from expected behavior is important. Signs of tissue deterioration in the mouth, unusual face and body movements, unfamiliar odors from the mouth and unusual expression in the eyes are some of the observable signs that some form of drug is being used.

Most adolescents who have experimented with drugs follow the pattern of "the crowd" in dress and behavior even though they may come for the regular checkup to "throw parents off the track" in an attempt to hide their habits. If symptoms are recognized and conditions in the mouth seem to point toward the use of drugs, the situation must be referred to the dentist without any suggestion to the patient that symptoms have been noticed.

Prevention is again the key word. Stress certain good health habits that may overcome the desire for experimentation. While we are told not to preach but to find some other means of reaching adolescents, we must still depend on facts that will counteract the efforts of a sick society that beckons them to experimentation and eventual addiction. Subjects to stress in a positive manner are as follows:

personal cleanliness, good appearance and the social advantage of a fine set of teeth in a healthy mouth;

the importance of an adequate diet, *eaten regularly,* for good health, good complexion and good teeth;

restriction of sugars, particularly in place of protein, minerals, whole grains and vitamins;

the high incidence of dental decay at this age and how it can be offset by regular dental care and good personal hygiene.

The health educator's ability, creativity and ingenuity will be taxed to the utmost in meeting the challenge of educating the adolescent to resist the influence of experimentation. The adolescent can be influenced to believe in his own ability to cope with the stresses of growing up without the use of drugs.

Misconceptions Concerning Dental Treatment

Most erroneous opinions concerning dental treatment may be attributed to the lack of understanding of the nature of dental disease, its prevention and correction. Like many superstitions in our culture, much of the suspicion which has surrounded dental treatment is disappearing as larger segments of the population are exposed to dental health instruction in the dental office, in the schools and through the press. However, misunderstanding still persists and tends to confuse even the well-informed. Through intelligent communication, opinions can be changed before they become well-established fears that lead to undesirable reactions.

Teeth are Expendable. Dental treatment is not a luxury. It is necessary for good health. However, there are people who still believe that teeth are not expected to last a lifetime. One survey revealed that more than one-half of the respondents believed that "some people are just born with good teeth and others are not; there is not much anyone can do about it." A smaller but still significant group agreed that "no matter how well you take care of your teeth, eventually you will lose them."*

Treatment Procedures. There are so many fallacies about dental treatment that only a few can be discussed to indicate the extent of the problem. A commonly heard comment is, "John had only a small cavity in his tooth but when the dentist filled it there was a very large filling." The parent had not been told that all infected tooth structure around the cavity had to be removed to prevent recurrence of decay and that the cavity must be properly shaped to hold the filling material. Other examples of fallacies about dental treatment follow.

"Once a tooth is filled it is safe from decay." If the filling falls out due to extreme pressure or if recurrence of decay due to poor mouth hygiene causes the filling to break down, the dentist is blamed. Patients must be told that fillings and other types of restorations are not permanent cures but must be checked at frequent intervals with X rays and clinical inspections.

"I want to have them all out." No patient should be allowed to sacrifice teeth because he does not want to undergo dental treatment and the cost involved. He should be told that there are no real substitutes for his own teeth. The attitude of neglecting the teeth until they cannot be saved may

have deeper psychological implications. Some effort should be made to find out why the patient is unconsciously avoiding dental treatment.

"I do not want X rays taken. I am afraid of the radiation." This observation has been mentioned before in the text but it bears repetition. Suffice it to say that every patient that needs X rays should also know that it is a safe and necessary procedure.

"I have heard that teeth are worn away by frequent cleanings." A great many fallacies exist about the regular cleaning of teeth, especially about scaling below the free margin of the gingiva. The patient should know the importance of regular professional prophylaxis in the prevention of dental caries and the onset of periodontal disease. Patients should understand that prophylaxis is not a cosmetic treatment or a means of increasing the dentist's income, but a vital part of good dental health. Deposits on teeth are not nature's way of protecting teeth, but the principal cause of tooth decay and periodontal disease. In the treatment, the gingiva is not forced away from the teeth, but by removing the irritating deposits and plaque, inflammation is reduced and the tone of the gingival tissue is restored so that with proper home care the soft tissues will cling more closely to the teeth. Prophylaxis is a preventive service that is given at designated intervals to assure good dental health.

"I use an advertised mouthwash but I still have halitosis." A statement of this kind brings into action all the knowledge we have concerning the claims of advertisers. It is an excellent opportunity to instruct the patient about the actual value of a mouthwash and the transient effect it has on the breath. More halitosis is caused by accumulations of debris on the teeth and poor mouth hygiene than by systemic causes. A toothbrush and a slightly abrasive dentifrice are needed to remove these accumulations.

Past Dental Experiences. Patients are conditioned for or against dental treatment

* Young, W. O., Striffler, D. E.: THE DENTIST, HIS PRACTICE AND HIS COMMUNITY, W. B. Saunders Co., Philadelphia, 1964, p. 192.

by their past experiences. Some of the factors which cause adverse attitudes are pain and discomfort in the dental chair, the amount and type of dental service required and the unpleasant after-effects of treatment. Whether or not the patient accepts preventive dental services depends largely upon how he has been conditioned to expect recall at specified intervals. He must be convinced that regular checkups will eliminate pain and the loss of teeth. A considerable amount of persuasion must be used over a long period of time in order to accomplish this goal. People change only when they are convinced that the change has specific benefit for them.

Concerning Nutrition and Dental Health. The amount of misinformation concerning nutrition and diet in reference to general health is appalling even among informed people. Our teen-agers suffer from malnutrition in an affluent society. Nutritional counseling has been recognized as a neglected area of education in our schools. Although it is difficult to find convincing evidence that poor nutrition affects teeth directly, there are indications that good general health depends on an adequate diet throughout life. The reduction of free sugar in the American diet has not yet been effectively accomplished.

Turner says, "Another misconception some people have is that there is need for some *refined sugar* in the daily diet. Many natural foods contain sugar, (the kind that does not decay teeth) along with other nutrients. Sugar supplies only calories. Many people would be more adequately nourished if fewer calories were eaten in the form of refined sugars."* And we might add, there would be fewer cavities.

There is agreement among scientists that "a tooth for every child" is a fallacy. Calcium cannot be withdrawn from teeth once they have been formed, yet many believe

that the unborn child absorbs calcium from the teeth of the mother.

The loss of teeth during pregnancy is due in part to poor mouth hygiene. Pregnant women avoid brushing their teeth because of nausea. They avoid dental treatment for the same reason. Neglect causes rampant caries during gestation and immediately after the birth of the child. This condition can be avoided if proper toothbrushing is taught and practiced during pregnancy. More frequent prophylaxis and x-ray examinations are usually advised.

In the first part of this text an effort has been made to consider the education and instruction of the individual from the point of view of the psychological, biological and social forces that affect his total health and, in particular, his dental health. The next section will be concerned with dental health education in the community.

Questions for Review and Discussion

1. What are the aims of the "educative moment" in dental practice?

2. Discuss the two philosophies of patient education in the dental office. Which do you prefer? Why?

3. What is meant by a chairside personality? Name several attributes.

4. Write out instructions for home care for a patient who has just had his first dental prophylaxis.

5. Make a list of questions patients have asked you in the last week during dental prophylaxis. Discuss these and tell how you answered them.

6. What is the dental hygienist's role in the instruction of the denture patient?

7. What visual aids would you use in instructing a patient in mouth hygiene? Be creative in your selection.

8. How did you control the last case of fear in a child whom you treated?

9. Children need special consideration when they are given dental appointments. State some precautions that should be observed.

10. A child may learn a number of basic

---

* Turner, C. E.: PERSONAL AND COMMUNITY HEALTH, 11th. Edition, C. V. Mosby Co., St. Louis, 1959, p. 51.

dental health concepts while he is being treated. What are they?

11. Explain the misconcept "teeth are expendable."

12. What can the dental hygienist do about recognizing a drug habit in a patient during dental prophylaxis?

13. Discuss the symptoms of drug abuse that may be found in the mouth. Use collateral reading for this assignment.

14. Add to the dental fallacies discussed in the text with those you have heard during clinical practice.

15. Make a "picture a page" book for use in a dental office.

16. Discuss the following statement: "Patients need not be informed about nutrition in our culture. What they really need is to stop eating so much."

17. Convince a patient that his teeth are a valuable part of his body and as such should be preserved throughout life.

18. What is meant by "persuasion"?

Selected Readings

Bates, R. S.: THE FINE ART OF UNDERSTANDING PATIENTS, Medical Economics Book Division, Oradell, N. J., 1968.

Collett, H. A.: "Influence of Dentist-Patient Relationship on Attitudes and Adjustment to Dental Treatment," Journal American Dental Association, October, 1969, p. 879.

Taylor, L. S.: "Xrays and the Dental Profession," Journal American Dental Association, October, 1969, p. 885.

PART II

DENTAL HEALTH EDUCATION IN COMMUNITY HEALTH PROGRAMS

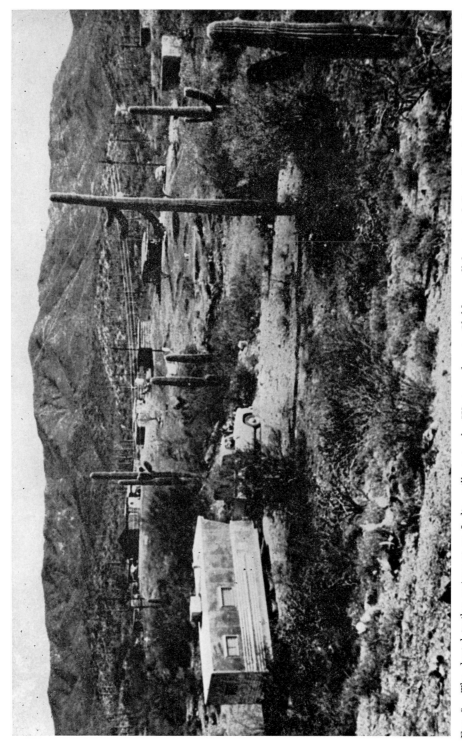

Fig. 6.—The dental trailer arrives at an Indian village in the Western desert. Children will be treated first, then the adults with acute problems, and then restorative dentistry will be made available to those who require it. (Courtesy, Indian Health Service, Dental Branch, U.S. Public Health Service, Department of Health, Education and Welfare.)

Chapter 5

Dental Disease—A Public Health Problem

It is important to the individual to possess a sufficient store of sound health knowledge that can be called upon as the basis for good judgement and desirable decisions regarding individual, family and community health. It is difficult for an individual to acquire and maintain a suitable level of knowledge about health without learning basic information during school years. Such knowledge must be continually reinforced and updated through exposure to an effective program of community health education.

Health knowledge is not an end in itself. What we are mainly concerned with are health practices and what the individual does when he is confronted with the necessity of making a decision on a matter involving his health.

Health education in the community deals primarily with the psychosocial environment, that is, the attitude exhibited by individuals and groups toward a particular practice. Drug abuse is a startling example. Ten years ago it was socially unacceptable and addicts were only a few members of some subcultural groups. Today the growth in drug use can be traced directly to one major factor, *the drastic change in the psychosocial environment*. The attitude toward the use of drugs, particularly among adolescents in many cultural groups, has been drastically altered in a matter of a few short years from total rejection to virtual acceptance.

How does this situation affect dental health in the community? It demonstrates the fact that dental health education must strive to become a part of a complete system of health education in the home, in the schools and in the community. It must be made socially acceptable, or rather, *socially expected behavior* not only in the middle and upper classes but also in disadvantaged groups. Health habits and attitudes can be changed through education when they become socially acceptable in a society.

The Total Problem of Dental Care

A survey of 915 white children between 18 and 39 months of age showed that at 23 months the children did not have cavities. From the twenty-third to the thirty-ninth month 57.2% had developed cavities. The average number of d.e.f. teeth at 39 months was 4.65. The survey indicates the prevalence of dental caries in the youngest group of preschool children.[*]

During the school life, all children will need some form of dental treatment. At best 1 to 2% of the school population will escape the ravages of dental disorders. The amount of dental treatment needed by an individual is determined first by the

[*] Hennon, K. H., Stookey, G. K., Muhler, J. C.: "Prevalence and Distribution of Dental Caries in Preschool Children," Journal American Dental Association, December, 1969, p. 1405.

41

severity of the attack upon his teeth and second by the amount of treatment that he has already received. Accumulated dental needs due to neglect over a period of time require more treatment time than regular semiannual visits to the dentist when all dental treatment has been completed.

It is estimated that 180 million persons in this country have accumulated more than 700 million unfilled cavities. To repair these teeth would require a minimum of six hours of dentist-time per person. The amount of dental treatment time available now is less than one hour per person per year. The magnitude of the problem of dental health on a community basis is almost incomprehensible. Research shows that males have greater need for dental services than females; the poor need more service than the financially able; Negroes need more service than whites and the uneducated need more service than the educated. Since dental disease is progressive and cumulative, the amount of dental service required increases with age.

The numerous dental problems of low-income families are apparent in the National Nutrition Survey of 1969 conducted in low-income areas of Texas, Kentucky, New York and Louisiana by the United States Public Health Service. Throughout the country the average adult has 5.7 filled teeth and 1.2 decayed teeth. People from the survey areas have 6.3 decayed teeth and only 1.0 filled teeth. The survey found that 92.6% of the people in the survey had one or more carious teeth which needed filling or extraction; 90% of the children under the age of 17, and 97% of all young adults were in need of filling, extractions or both. Nearly half of all the persons with teeth were victims of periodontal disease. Beginning with 10% of children under 10 years of age, the percentage of persons with periodontal problems increased rapidly. At ages 10 to 16 about 35% were affected; at ages 17 to 24 about 50% showed periodontal involvement.

Total Expenditures for Dental Care

Each year the U.S. Department of Commerce estimates consumer expenditures for various goods and services. The statistics include a long-term series of data on dental health and medical care.

In 1968, a total 38 billion, five hundred eight million dollars were spent on health care. Three billion, five hundred fifty million of this amount was spent for dental care. From 1966 through 1968 the amount spent for dental care exceeded the total amount spent for medical care for 1935 and 1940. This is attributed to the constantly increasing population, a prosperous economy, increased appreciation of dental health and general inflation which has reduced the purchasing power of the dollar by slightly more than 60% since 1939. Yet dentistry's portion of the health dollar has declined from 13.9% in 1940 to 9.2% in 1968.*

Basic Concepts of Demand and Supply as Applied to Dental Treatment

The *demand* for health services, curative or preventive, must be distinguished from the *need* for these services. Many persons have physical defects of which they are unaware. Others, even though they recognize these defects, do not seek care because of ignorance, inaccessible services, fear of expense or psychological inhibitions. An individual's need for treatment can be discovered and appraised by health inspections and examinations, but the actual *demand* for treatment will depend on his recognition of his need for it, upon his financial resources and upon the accessibility of care.

The *need* for preventive service is practically universal, but *demand* arises only as a result of education. The chief aim of dental health education is to develop knowledge of the values of various preven-

* "Expenditures and Prices for Dental and Other Health Care," Report of Councils and Bureaus, Journal American Dental Association, December, 1969, p. 1447.

tive and curative services and to encourage a demand for service which corresponds to the need. The demand for dental care has increased each year. Greatly accelerated demand is expected for the next ten years because there is a continuing increase of interest in dental health due to education, increase in family income and better methods of financing dental care by prepayment and insurance plans.

The individual must make choices among dentists and other resources such as clinics of various types when he seeks care. The right of free choice among dental treatment resources is nevertheless restricted by many practical conditions. They are as follows: 1. the geographical availability of treatment; 2. the need for services of specialists in dentistry; 3. financial restrictions; 4. limitations of patient's knowledge of location, qualifications, personality and charges of dentists. The patient's freedom to do what he wishes is also limited by his knowledge of what he needs. The more numerous and complex the resources among which he may choose, the more knowledge he will need to make the best choice.

A great deal has been said about creating demands for treatment that cannot be met in reality because of shortages in dental manpower and facilities. It is particularly apparent among school children whose parents are willing to obtain treatment but find it unavailable. This dilemma is in the nature of an unmet need. It is not unique to dental treatment; it exists also in medical care and educational facilities. There is no validity to the argument that knowledge of dental needs should be withheld until facilities and manpower are available. Unless people become informed there is little hope that increased facilities for treatment will be developed.

Parents, educators, dentists and interested citizens should make the need known. They can stimulate interest in fulfilling the demand by encouraging the establishment of new facilities for treatment and by stimulating the efficient use of those which

already exist. The public grows more dentally conscious with each visit to the dentist. Marginal groups who cannot pay for dental care increase their demand for it every time they visit a clinic. When the *demand* for dental care decreases, dental *needs* pile up and expand beyond the demand. When the chance of obtaining dental service becomes remote, the group in low-income brackets loses interest and the demand drops off because of the fatalistic attitude that nothing can be done. A disturbing observation is that the *rate of utilization* is usually below the need among low-income groups where dental services are available without charge, *if no special health education* is given in the community, before and during treatment.

An effective program of dental health education in the schools must be reinforced by an active dental health education effort for adults at the community level. Failure to provide such a program may be costly to the individual and to the community in terms of poor dental health and low productivity. Upon this premise community dental health programs will be explored.

Standards of Adequate Services Within the Community

In "Suggested School Health Policies," a report by the National Education Association, it has been stated that community action sometimes is necessary in developing resources to meet the needs of all children. Leadership for such action should be provided cooperatively by the local medical and dental societies and the public health department. If community facilities for physical care appear inadequate, their extension should be recommended. If a community finds its local resources inadequate to meet the demonstrated need it may seek help from voluntary organizations or from county, state or federal agencies. This statement makes it clear that schools assume no responsibility for remedial treatment of school children.

Financial Support of Dental Care Programs

Dental services are financed in four ways, as follows: 1. Through fees paid by the individual when services are rendered. The largest amount of dental treatment is financed in this way through the efforts of the family. 2. Taxation as a means of paying for medical and dental care serves to distribute the financial burden over society as a whole. Persons receiving care pay for it only partly or indirectly. It is the method which departments of health and welfare use to provide dental care. 3. Dental fees may be paid for by charity. When dentists reduce their fees for children of large families or for "borderline cases" not entitled to welfare, they are providing a charity service. Charity also takes the form of monetary gifts from individuals, philanthropic organizations and other nongovernment bodies. They usually support clinics and constitute but a small part of the whole picture of dental care. 4. Prepayment plans for dental care in which groups of people make periodic prepayments of fixed amounts so that dental fees will be paid by an insurance company similar to Blue Cross.

Prepayment Plans for Dental Treatment

So many people are covered by hospital and medical insurance that there is a tendency for more of them to seek further protection by budgeting for dental care as well. Most prepayment plans allow the individual free choice of a dentist. A dentist may or may not participate in the plan, as he chooses. The dentist receives a fee for each service from a predetermined schedule of fees. This type of plan is known as "open panel." Treatment is given in the private dental office.

The "closed panel" prepayment plan does not allow free choice of a dentist. The patient must accept the dentist assigned to him. Dentists are hired as salaried employees and usually treat patients in clinics equipped and maintained by the parent organization. Labor unions, industrial groups and some paid health services use this method. Because dentistry is such a personal service, involving a rapport between dentist and patient, there has been some resentment toward the closed panel system.

The dental profession has attempted to preserve the dentist-patient relationship by organizing community-wide groups of people insured by dental service corporations sponsored by the American Dental Association but organized under state dental societies. The first dental service corporation was organized in the State of Washington in 1954. The National Association of Dental Service Plans was incorporated as a nonprofit national coordinating agency in January 1965 by the American Dental Association. For expediency, the name was changed in 1969 to the Delta Dental Plan, with the symbol of two triangles imposed within a square. Each state plan will use this symbol so that it will be recognized as the one accepted and sponsored by the American Dental Association. Among the prepaid plans are (1) dental service corporations (Delta Plans); (2) commercial insurance companies; (3) group practice or clinics; (4) nonprofit insurance corporations; and (5) union-financed plans paid by union dues or other union resources. Among the union and industrial plans are five differently financed types: (1) plans financed by employees by withholding fees from salaries; (2) employer-employee financed plans in which each party pays a share; (3) employer-financed plan commonly known as a fringe benefit; (4) union-employed plan in which each party finances a share of the costs; and (5) union-financed plans paid through union dues and other union income.

Prepaid dental care is probably the most widely discussed employee benefit in management and labor circles. A huge national market for health care benefits has turned its attention to dental care as the next addition to the employee benefit package.

The implications of this breakthrough and the demand for programs and services that it will generate will affect dental service corporations administrating and underwriting the programs.

There are twenty-seven active state Delta Plans and more to come. Approximately two million Americans are provided with prepaid dental care coverage. Some 391 private group contracts are in force and 179 contracts involving publicly funded programs. The summary of the dental service plans is shown in Table 1. To realize the extent to which the Delta Dental Plan contributes to the dental welfare of the population, consider the California Delta Dental Plan with a total enrollment of approximately 1.6 million people. It is presently administrating 280 separate privately and publicly funded dental care programs and last year paid out more than $31 million for dental care benefits on behalf of its subscribers.

In conclusion, it is apparent that the prepayment plans for dental treatment will continue to increase and that the demand for dental services will continue to rise in proportion to the increase in number of

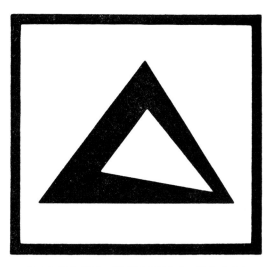

A DELTA DENTAL PLAN

Table 1. Summary of Dental Service Plan Programs as of December 31, 1968.

Programs (by category)	No. of programs	No. of subscribers
PRIVATE		
Underwritten	373	1,449,613
Administered on cost-plus basis	18	17,862
Total	391	1,467,475
PUBLIC		
Head Start	149	37,874
Follow Through	1	75
Upward Bound	1	105
Community Action	7	1,806
Child and Youth Care	1	250
Job Corps	2	260
Public Assistance (State)	1	149,355
Public Assistance (County)	1	225
Maternal and Infant Care	3	630
Office of Education	2	329
Office of Education (Title I)	3	350
Children's Bureau: PRESCAD,	2	50,000
Neighborhood Youth Corps, Operation Summertime	3	
Department of Health		8,000
Title XIX	1	3,000
Neighborhood Health Center	2	300
private practice extension program	1	
Total	179	252,559
GRAND TOTAL: Private and public programs	570	1,720,034

plans. They provide a potent source of dental health education and the members will use the free services with increasing frequency. Children will probably benefit the most as their parents are motivated to the benefits of regular systematic dental care. It will take time to change the attitude of a generation of people toward dental care, but with the problem of paying dental fees out of pocket removed, the transition should be rapid.

Services Rendered by Public Agencies

The first program for medical care was established in 1798 by the United States Congress when it voted to establish the Marine Hospital Fund for merchant seamen. The Marine Hospital was the forerunner of the United States Public Health Service. Health services provided by the federal government have expanded at a steady rate from this beginning. The increase has expanded the scope of the services and the number of eligible groups treated. A number of factors have contributed to this growth: (a) changing attitudes of large segments of the population in regard to health, (b) change of economic status of minority groups who demand services for which they are unable to pay, (c) increase in the amount of scientific knowledge available for the treatment and prevention of disease, (d) the altruistic attitude by individuals and government of caring for those unable to care for themselves, and (e) the protection and welfare of the population at large.

Dentistry did not enter into the public health services until 1919. As the nature of health problems changed from combating communicable disease to attaining the maximum potential for productive living for all, the change from emergency relief of pain and repair of defects to prevention of dental disease and the protection of tooth structure has occurred. Public interest has increased, not only in providing services but also in making available programs of instruction and education for better dental health practices.

Functions of Government in Dental Health

The federal government provides dental care directly to the largest group of citizens, military personnel and their dependents, through the various branches of the armed forces.

The United State Public Health Service, a branch of the Department of Health, Education and Welfare, provides services for merchant seamen, the U. S. Coast Guard, American Indians, Alaskan natives and inmates of federal prisons. The Veterans Administration provides dental services to veterans. All patients in veteran hospitals receive complete dental care and dental health instruction. Medicare and Medicaid under social security provide limited dental services to the aged and the indigent through direct payment for services rendered by the dentist.

In order to keep the mainstream of services in the state and local communities the federal government provides funds through a system of grants-in-aid. For each dollar the state is required to provide the federal government provides two dollars. These grants are awarded to the states, which in turn distribute needed funds to local communities.

No effort has been made to list all the government services that include some kind of dental program because these are constantly changing. The intent is to list only the principal services to provide an overall view of the extent of these services.

Functions of the States in Dental Care

Each state administers its public health and welfare according to the needs of its population. Public dental care programs differ widely from state to state as to functions and the sections of the population covered by these services. In the main, states provide dental care to prisoners and inmates of state hospitals; to crippled children, to welfare patients and to aged indigents. There is a distinction between the work of the department of public health, which is mainly concerned with helping people to help themselves and promoting community health, and the department of welfare, which is concerned mainly with meeting the immediate needs of those who do not have the minimum necessities for healthful living.

In all these programs the department in charge of dental services exerts leadership in setting standards, in promoting quality of services and in promoting efficient use of resources through well-rounded programs of dental health education. The state may provide the financial support for the program of dental health education, but it must be conducted on the local community level to be effective.

Dental Programs Under Department of Welfare

Dental health is an expanding area of service in local communities, particularly for children. From time to time directives concerning these services are issued by welfare departments. A recent release defines what services shall be provided for children. They are, in brief:

1. All children shall have clinical examinations, including bite-wing x-ray examination, by a dentist every six months.

2. Orthodontic treatment shall be provided when a dental problem is considered to be a physical handicap.

3. Complete, adequate and high-quality dental care shall be provided for all persons under the care of the department.

4. Fees shall be based on a schedule provided by the department of welfare and an appropriate advisory group.

5. All dentists should be encouraged to participate in the service; there shall be a free choice of dentists by welfare recipients where fee-for-service plans operate.

It is apparent that all children under the care of the department of welfare are en-

titled to adequate dental treatment. The problem is to persuade parents to request this aid and then to check the children so that dental appointments are kept and the necessary treatment completed. The school has a valid responsibility to see that all children on welfare receive the services to which they are entitled even though parents do not request these services. It is often possible for school personnel (nurses and dental hygienists) to contact the case workers. They are most cooperative and have considerable influence with parents. Often parents are unaware of the services available or they are reticent to ask for more aid, fearing that it might reduce their meager allowances.

The *medically indigent* are those families that have sufficient income to provide food, clothing and shelter but who lack funds for medical and dental services. In many cases they are entitled to aid under welfare laws. It is suggested that all possible sources of treatment be explored by health personnel, particularly for school children. Many sources for dental treatment are unknown and unused.

Dental Health Education in Nursing Homes

Dental care for the aged and chronically ill in nursing homes and extended-care facilities is a problem that is receiving more attention at present although it has existed for a number of years. The dental aspect of patient care is slighted because of lack of funds, lack of personnel and lack of interest on the part of administrators and workers. They do not recognize the need for good mouth hygiene even in edentulous patients. Relief of pain has heretofore been the goal of treatment and nothing has been done to instruct patients in their own responsibility for mouth cleanliness.

The House of Delegates of the American Dental Association, recognizing the need for such education, adopted a statement developed by the Council on Dental Health in 1969. The recommendations were drafted for the guidance of advisory dentists to the Medicare facilities, but they also apply to dental personnel working in nursing homes or other long-term care institutions.

"Institutions participating in Medicare are required to,

1. obtain the services of an *Advisory Dentist*

2. to assist patients to obtain regular and emergency dental care.

Advisory dentists should make recommendations in the following areas: provision of emergency dental services, mechanisms to provide needed dental treatment, policies on oral hygiene, co-ordination of services with medical, nursing and other staff, and training staff to assist patients in proper oral hygiene. Dentists will be remunerated by Medicare for their advisory responsibilities. Remuneration for other services would be on a fee-for-service or other acceptable basis."* The continuing oral hygiene program in nursing homes should be based on the following principles.

1. All patients should have a dental examination after admission.

2. Periodic evaluations should be made, with particular attention to the detection of possible malignant lesions.

3. Dental treatment should be provided according to the physical and psychological ability of the patient. The dentist should be informed of any physical or mental limitations.

4. Whenever possible the treatment should be performed by the patient's own dentist.

5. The staff should be instructed to be alert to any changes in the patient's oral health status.

6. Consultation should be provided on diet and nutrition.

7. All staff should be given dental health

* "Providing Dental Care in Nursing Homes," Council on Dental Health, Journal American Dental Association, January, 1970, p. 152.

instruction and should be taught to assist patients in practicing recommended daily oral hygiene procedures.

Dental hygienists can be valuable assistants in the effective operation of the dental programs in nursing homes. They can assist the dentist in providing treatment, teach patients how to maintain good mouth hygiene and provide dental health information to the staff members in workshops and conferences at the local and state levels.

Special Services for the Handicapped

There are children and adults in our society who are incapable of using the usual toothbrushes, dental floss and other aids to mouth health due to physical, mental and emotional handicaps. The destructive effects of poor dental hygiene have been documented, particularly for the individual with cerebral palsy. The poor dental hygiene is due to difficulty in toothbrushing; the inability of the person to clean his own mouth because of muscular spasms and tremors. These individuals are prone to gagging and vomiting when a brush is placed in the mouth. There is failure of the tongue, cheeks, lips and saliva to clean the mouth as in normal individuals. These individuals have a high rate of dental decay and a high incidence of gingival disease. Many of the mentally retarded cannot coordinate the mental and muscular action in order to brush their teeth and must therefore rely on others to do the task or to take long, painstaking periods of instruction and practice with them. The incidence of dental caries and gingival disorders increases in direct proportion to the severity of physical handicap.

The answer seems to lie in providing extensive dental health instruction on a person-to-person basis using specially designed devices unique to each individual. Many such devices have been made by creative dentists, dental hygienists and industrial designers and are being produced commercially. The brushes vary in shape and handle angulation. Some are smaller than usual, others have much larger handles. Electric brushes work well in some cases.

Research is being conducted on a chewable device which has a handle that the patient can hold while chewing on a semi-hard rubber sponge. This device not only cleans the teeth when it is being chewed but also supplies the exercise needed in the absence of coarse foods which these patients cannot chew. The mechanical scrubbing action massages and stimulates circulation in the soft tissues. Instruction in the use of the device is essential.*

Motivation is the key to success, and fortunately, handicapped individuals are very anxious to learn anything that will add to their limited abilities. Patience, kindness, empathy and a real sense of liking them are the best means to stimulate the handicapped to practice good mouth hygiene.

Project Head Start: Implications for Community Dental Health

The Head Start program for preschool children from underprivileged homes started through legislation in 1965 as part of the Office of Economic Opportunity. During the summer of 1966, 575,000 children had been exposed to a dental examination either by a dentist or at least a dental hygienist. Approximately 600 year-round and follow-through programs had enrolled 193,000 children in 1968. A report in 1970 indicates that 2,000 communities have some interest in the Head Start program. It has been estimated that since its beginning the project has reached 5% of the population under 5 years of age. Each of the children involved has been given at least one visit to the dentist; 85% of the children enrolled suffer from dental diseases as compared to 12% who have various medical problems.

The programs are financed in a number of ways. Some large cities such as New York, Detroit and Washington, D.C. have shown that the health department as an administrator can either provide direct service to children or delegate the provision of service through the private dental office, directly or through the dental service corporations (Delta Plans). In some instances communities have provided equipment and buildings in their budgets. Private organizations, through volunteer services, have given hours of time to these programs. Dental schools have provided clinical services and the United States Navy has accepted responsibility for providing a preventive dentistry program for those dependents' children who would otherwise fall into the Head Start bracket.

For the first time real interest has been concentrated on the preschool age child. An intense interest in dental health has been generated through recruiting neighborhood parents in the program. Volunteers, aides and neighborhood workers have assisted parents in taking children to dental offices or clinics. Communication thus established has given motivation to parents to seek dental care for their children.

The program has gone beyond the usual school inspection program and is attempting to provide complete dental care wherever possible. This fact met with some resistance from the dental profession until it was pointed out that fee-for-service would be part of the financial arrangement and that the community-backed program would add to the prestige of dentists who accepted Head Start patients. In summary the experience of the Head Start program indicates that

1. preschool deprived children have unique dental health problems;
2. there is a shift of emphasis from dental inspection to treatment of defects;
3. not only the children but the parents and health professionals receive instruction in dental health procedures;
4. mobilization of community resources has increased the efficiency of the program;
5. involvement of local residents, includ-

* Holcomb, F. H., Taylor, P. P., Saunders, W. A.: "Comparison of Oral Hygiene Devices for the Handicapped," *Journal of Dentistry for Children,* July-August, 1970. p. 325.

ing parents, volunteers, social workers and others has spread the word for better dental health among a greater segment of the underprivileged. The Head Start program, if it is continued at an efficient level, should reduce the need for extensive dental care by treating defects as they occur in young children. Tooth structure will be saved and less treatment time will be necessary during the succeeding school years.

Questions for Review and Discussion

1. Explain the psychosocial implications of the environment upon the dental health of a community. What efforts can be made to improve dental health at this level?

2. It has been estimated that to give the whole population complete dental treatment would require six dentist-hours per person per year. At the present time less than one hour per person is available per year. Enumerate some efforts that could be suggested to provide more care per person in the population (thought question).

3. Explain the concept of supply and demand as applied to dental health.

4. Name the four methods of financing dental treatment.

5. What is the main difference between "open panel dentistry" and "closed panel dentistry"?

6. What are the Delta Plans for financing dental treatment?

7. Explain the function of grants-in-aid provided by the United States government in reference to dental services.

8. Look up the provisions of Medicare nd Medicaid that are concerned with den- tal services.

9. Define the term "medically indigent" is compared to the term "economically dis- dvantaged."

10. The American Dental Association recommends that all nursing homes and long-care institutions have an "advisory dentist." State the duties and responsibilities assigned to the dentist.

11. Handicapped individuals have spe- cific problems in obtaining good dental hygiene. State some of the conditions that need special attention. How are these dif- ficulties solved?

12. Visit the Head Start project in your vicinity and note the following for discus- sion in class: What services are rendered and by whom? Who is responsible for dental health instruction? Does this person have adequate training for teaching? How adequate is the instruction? Are there any dental hygienists involved? How many children are given dental treatment in this particular group? Are the dental records adequate and accurate? Do parents and other workers participate in the project? What can be done to improve the services in dental health?

Selected Readings

"A Unique Opportunity—Model Cities Program," Journal American Dental Association, August, 1969, p. 236.

Bowden, J. W.: "Dentistry's Role in Regional Medical Programs," American Journal of Public Health, May, 1970, p. 844.

"Dental Care for the Home Bound," Journal American Dental Association, July, 1969, p. 68.

"Delta Dental Plans," Journal American Dental Association, July, 1969, p. 55; August, 1969, p. 1074.

"Dental Health Program for American Indians, Eskimos and Aleuts," U.S. Dept. Health, Education and Welfare, Public Service Pub- lication, No. 1585, 1967.

Fisher, M. A.: "New Directions for Dentistry," Americal Journal of Public Health, May, 1970, p. 848.

Gillespie, G. M.: "Project Head Start and Dental Care—One Summer of Experience," Ameri- can Journal of Public Health, January, 1968, p. 90.

North, A. F.: "Project Head Start, Its Implications for School Health," American Journal of Public Health, April, 1970, p. 698.

Project Head Start Health Services, A Guide for Project Directors and Health Personnel, Washington, D.C., Office of Economic Op- portunity, 1967.

"Title XIX Children's Dental Care," Journal American Dental Association, June, 1969, p. 1277.

"Title XIX Medicaid," Journal American Dental Association, June, 1969, p. 1273.

Zapp, J. S.: "Dentistry, Legislation and the New Administration," American Journal of Public Health, May, 1970, p. 844.

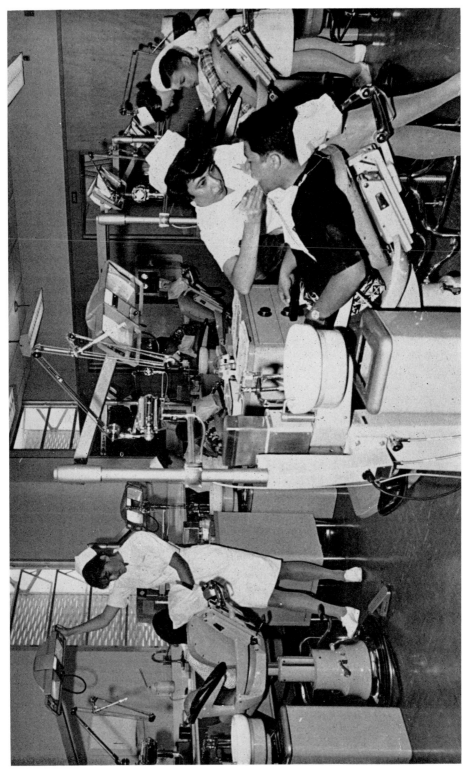

Fig. 7.—Medicaid Task Force recommends the inclusion of dental care for children from five to twelve years of age. Dental health clinics include treatment and instruction. (Courtesy, Department of Dental Hygiene, University of Hawaii.)

Chapter 6

Dental Treatment for All Children

Population Trends

The trends in population growth should be known and understood if the present and future dental health needs of the population are to be met. The Conference on Health Services for Children and Youth stated in brief that the population of the United States (200 million) is growing younger. Of the population, 50% are now under 25 years of age. The median age for whites has moved since 1955 from 31 to 25; from 29 to 22 for nonwhites.

Approximately 19 million children are under 5 years of age. The population over 60 years of age is also increasing. The age group in between, normally the source of support of the other groups, is relatively smaller in number and it is this section of society that is feeling the pressure of the costs of meeting the health needs of the elderly and the young.

The majority of children and youth as well as their parents has become city dwellers. Two-thirds of the young people under 20 live in or near metropolitan areas which cover only 1% of the land area, but contain 64% of the total population. Only 6% of white children and 8% of nonwhite children live on farms. Most of the increase in population of nonwhites has been in cities while the white population has increased in the suburbs.

By definition large families are those with 4 or more children. Of families with children under eighteen 11% are large, yet 39% (25 million) of children live in these large families.

There were 9 million children living in families with incomes under $3,000 in 1965. Another 43 million were in families with an income of $6,000, and 17 million in families with an income of $10,000 or more. Approximately 15 million children live in poverty. The majority of these are *white*. However, among nonwhite children over half live in poverty. Nine million white children and 6 million nonwhite children live in poverty at this time.

It is clear that social, cultural and economic circumstances influence the quality of medical and dental health care available to children and adolescents. Those at greatest risk, with the greatest need and the least health services are the nonwhite, the poor, the central city or rural dwellers, those living in families headed by one parent and those living in families with low educational backgrounds.

The primary sources which seem to exert major influence on the health services include uneven distribution of income, family disruption, uneven distribution of services, urban migration and the lack of a preventive approach in health services, especially for the young children.

Despite its vast resources, scientific knowledge and administrative skills, this country has not yet developed a national plan for the protection of children's health. A larger commitment and immediate mobilization of all technical, financial and social resources from private and public sectors are required to make high-quality health care available to all children. More complete application must be made of our knowledge from recent research, with emphasis on the requirements for optimal physical, psychological and intellectual growth of the children. Attention to necessities such as income, housing, food and education and their total effect upon child health is essential. Significant changes in the financing, organization and methods of delivery of health services must be made. The training and utilization of new types of health workers are imperative because of the serious shortage of professional personnel. Health workers must assume leadership to establish close cooperation between persons from related fields and consumers to work out solutions to dental health problems.*

Dental Treatment Needs of Children

All children will need some form of dental treatment during their school life. The most effective approach to dental care is to begin with the young child; correct the accumulated dental defects and recall the patient periodically for maintenance care. It has been shown that the time required for initial care for the repair of accumulated dental disease varies with age. Children seven years old require approximately two hours to correct accumulated defects and one hour of the dentist's time the following year for maintenance care. If the child reaches ten years of age before receiving dental treatment, he will require three hours of chair time to repair accumulated defects and slightly more than one hour for yearly maintenance. In clinical situations it has been estimated that during one year each dentist can take care of about 530 children requiring initial treatment of ac-

cumulated defects. This number increases to over 1,300 after maintenance care becomes established, and includes new cases that must have initial care. This type of program has been called an incremental dental care program.

If good dental health instruction is included in such a program there will be an added benefit. The lasting effect of instruction should result in establishing a positive attitude toward good dental health habits. It has been reported that children exposed to regular dental care in an organized community program tend to continue in the established pattern after leaving the program.

Supply and Demand Applied to Preventive Services

The concept of supply and demand has been discussed at length in Chapter 5 but certain aspects bear repeating as they apply to dental treatment for children. A child's need for treatment can be discovered and appraised by inspection and examinations. The actual demand for care depends largely on the attitude of his parents. The need for preventive services is practically universal but the demand increases only in proportion to the educative effort. The chief aim of dental health education is to develop knowledge and an understanding of the various preventive and curative services, thus creating the demand for these services that corresponds to the need.

Some school systems in large cities have operated dental clinics but with greater community awareness of the importance of dental health, the responsibility for providing dental treatment for needy children belongs to the community welfare and health agencies rather than the schools. Some states prohibit the use of school funds for any remedial treatment of students. As far back as 1949 the Federal Security Agency adopted the policy that parents have primary responsibility for the health of their children. Health programs

---

*"Conference on Health Services for Children and Youth, March, 1969" American Journal of Public Health, April, 1970.

should be designed to assist parents in discharging this responsibility but they should not assume it for them. Clinical facilities should not be set up in school buildings unless the school building is a community center and unless there is general agreement among local groups that such location provides the best solution for the specific community.

Standards for Tax-supported Dental Care for Indigent Children

The following statement of policy was adopted by the American Dental Association:

The program should stress rehabilitation and prevention.

There should be respect for the rights and dignity of the individual.

Information about the illness of patients should remain confidential.

Services should be organized for maximum economy without sacrificing quality of treatment.

Services should be rendered promptly. Emergency treatment may be given before eligibility is established.

Standards of eligibility should be applied without discrimination.

Financial eligibility for tax-supported care should be determined by a public agency.

These standards are an attempt to show that indigence is a respectable state in this society, that it carries no stigma, but that it is considered a temporary state of emergency, recognized and provided for by government aid. If this attitude is established in the minds of parents, the available services for dental care will be used to capacity. Stimulation must come from health personnel who are familiar with the need and cognizant of the social blocks that arise against accepting aid. One way of giving welfare families a new start is to provide their children with the best possible health care.

Standards of Dental Treatment for Children

The American Dental Association and Public Health Dentists are agreed that minimum standards of dental care for children are as follows:

1. Periodic examination, including X rays and prophylaxis.
2. Restoration of carious teeth with amalgam or silicate filling or with metal castings.
3. Pulp treatments, including cappings and partial or total pulpotomies.
4. Anesthesia, whenever it is necessary for the control of pain.
5. Preventive orthodontic appliances to maintain space and prevent malocclusion.
6. Prosthetic appliances to replace missing teeth in order to restore function and improve appearance.
7. Treatment of periodontal infection.
8. Extraction of diseased, impacted and supernumerary teeth.
9. Surgical procedures whenever they are necessary for the health of the child.
10. Education of the parent and the child to encourage the application of scientific knowledge for the prevention of disease and the promotion of health.

Release Time for Dental Appointments During School Hours

It is impossible to treat children only when they are not engaged in school activities because of the patient load each dentist must assume. Saturdays, holidays, and hours after school are not the best times for dental treatment of children because they conflict with the activities of the family or encroach on the child's play time. Usually children are tired after school and appointments at that time become unhappy experiences. If dental treatment is to be accepted children must be permitted to use school time in order to fulfill the expectations of the school health program. Release time for appointments during school hours has been discussed pro and con. Some agreement has been reached and the consensus is that children should be excused to keep dental appointments during school hours. Staggering the appointment hours prevents loss of class in any one hour of the school day. Release time is not excessive since most children under private dental care do not require more than two appointments each six months.

Dental appointments should be treated as excused, legal absences for the purpose of computing state aid on the grounds that such appointments are educative experiences. A definite form for release from school will make the administration of release time more efficient. The form shown in figure 8 requires three signatures, the parent's, the dentist's and the school administrator's. It also has space for the dentist to indicate the time spent in his office. Any abuses that might arise from dental appointments can be eliminated by use of an adequate release form.

Dental Health Counseling for Parents

Health counseling has become a highly skilled function of health workers. Formerly, when physical defects were found in children through school inspections and examinations, those responsible for followup procedures used a dictatorial attitude. They expected that when parents were told that certain aspects of the child's physical condition had to be corrected or that home routines were to be changed, the parents would, without question "do as they were told." If parents failed to accept the advice, they were considered uncooperative. *Parents have the sole right to decide what shall be done for their children.* They have the right to accept or reject suggestions; to decide whether the child shall have treatment and who shall give the treatment. The role of the dental health educator is to inform the parents of

Sample Form—School Excuse for Dental Appointment

_____has a dental appointment for necessary service on
(Name of Pupil)

                                                                A.M.
_____19_____at_____P.M.

This service cannot be satisfactorily rendered outside of school hours. Therefore, it will be appreciated if this pupil be permitted to keep the appointment as indicated above.

_____   _____
(Signature of School Principal)   (Signature of Parent)

                                                 A.M.   A.M.
_____was in my office from _____P.M. to _____P.M. on
(Name of Pupil)

_____, 19_____ to have dental work done.

                                                    _____
                                                          (Signature of Dentist)
(To be returned to the School Principal)

Reverse Side of Dental Excuse Form

The Iowa State Department of Health and the Iowa State Dental Society recommend that your school cooperate in this dental excuse plan making it possible for the children in your school to obtain necessary dental service. The Iowa State Department of Public Instruction urges each local school district to give the dental excuse plan serious consideration.

A permit from school for such purpose, used judiciously, will enable school children to secure necessary dental service which cannot be satisfactorily rendered during the hours when school is not in session.

Fig. 8.—Reproduced from "Handbook of Dental Health Education," Bureau of Dental Hygiene, State University and State Board of Health of Iowa, p. 47.

the need; to interpret the facts so that parents understand what they are expected to do; to encourage them to accept the responsibility; to provide them with suggestions that will help them to obtain dental care; and finally, to *motivate* the parents to seek treatment that will give the child better dental health.

There is no doubt that most parents are deeply interested in the health and welfare of their children. At most 5 to 10% are known as "problem parents" who for a number of reasons may appear to neglect their children. Usually there is a good reason. It is the duty of the dental health educator to find the reason and to help solve the difficulty. What we are prone to call neglect is frequently failure on the part of parents to recognize the child's need for dental treatment. They do not realize the serious consequences of poor dental health. They are reticent in asking for help in order to comply with what the school expects. *Demonstrated cases of child neglect are matters for the courts.*

All efforts to bring the parents closer to the school life of the child should be reassuring and without false standards of perfection. Parents should be made to feel satisfaction and self-confidence in their ability to rear their children properly. The school must accept the socioeconomic level of the parents and through understanding and interest bring them by a process of education to accept voluntarily those principles of child behavior and development which the school has found to be best for each individual child.

If families are to change their attitudes and practices for better dental health, the school and the community must work directly with the parents and not expect children to act as health missionaries. Parents can be assisted to understand their responsibilities and to build a kind of relationship that will enable them to carry out functions that should be "family centered."

These are strong arguments for dental health conferences with parents. On occa-sion there have been objections to interfering with family privacy by requiring too many meetings with parents. The case for good dental health has suffered rather severely from this point of view. The authors' experience has shown that when nurses, health educators, classroom teachers or others interview parents in school or by a home visit, dental health problems must give way to more serious health problems. Parents are emotionally able to understand and cope with one health problem at a time. Any problem brought to their attention by the school is immediately magnified and emotionally charged. If dental health advice is necessary it should be provided in an atmosphere of relaxed friendliness by a qualified dental health educator. It should never be treated as an "emergency" if parents are to assume the right attitude toward preventive measures, regular dental care, mouth cleanliness and diet control. Even though the loss of a tooth may be imminent, pressuring the parents into immediate action is a poor approach to a continuous program of dental health in the home. Even a toothache can be a means of obtaining dental treatment for a child if he is sent home while he is in pain and thus indirectly showing the parents that the need is urgent. *A toothache should never be treated in school!* If the school nurse places eugenol-soaked cotton in a child's cavity and stops the pain, the parent does not see the child in pain and concludes that the school has taken care of the dental problem. They do not understand that such emergency treatment is not a cure. They assume that if the school practices this procedure it must be acceptable.

Most school laws require that parents be notified in writing of remediable defects. Printed forms have been devised for this purpose (Fig. 9). They generally provide for action on the part of the parent in that a section of the form is to be filled out by the dentist. The form indicates that the child is being treated, has completed dental treatment, or is in need of no treatment at

REPORT OF SCHOOL DENTAL INSPECTION

Parent or guardian_____

A dental inspection of your child _____ has been

made. This inspection shows:

☐ 1. Need for dental attention. It is recommended that your family dentist be consulted as

soon as possible.

☐ 2. No readily apparent dental defects. However, it is recommended that your child visit

your family dentist for a more complete examination.

_____   _____
DATE   SIGNED

CERTIFICATE OF DENTAL WORK DONE

This is to certify that the bearer:

☐ 1. Has had all necessary dental work completed.

☐ 2. Is under dental treatment.

☐ 3. Is in need of no dental work at this time.

Further recommendation _____

_____

_____   _____
DATE   SIGNATURE OF DENTIST

P L E A S E   R E T U R N   T H I S   C A R D   T O   T H E   T E A C H E R

FIG. 9.—Suggested form of dental report to be sent to parents after a dental inspection has been given in school.

this time. In the majority of cases the form is all that is needed to obtain action, *if the school dental health program is understood by the parents.*

Suggested Steps in Conducting Parent Conferences

The method of inviting the parent to school or requesting a visit to the home should be informal and friendly, not demanding. All available information concerning the child, including the general health record, the dental health record and the observations of the teacher should be read and at least the dental health record should be available during the conference.

The room in which the parent is received should be comfortable and attractive. If it is the health suite, there should be a comfortable chair. The dental health educator acting as a counselor should not sit behind a desk, but rather, in a chair similar to the one offered the parent. Interruptions should be avoided at all cost. If record of the visit is to be taped, the parent should be informed and his consent obtained. If a written record is to be made, as few notes as possible should be made during the interview. The report should be written after the parent has left. After rapport has been established by a short friendly conversation, the parent should be

---

TO THE PARENT: Our school has a health program that is designed to improve, protect and promote the health of the child. As a part of this health program we strongly urge all parents to have their children visit their dentist at least once a year for a dental examination and whatever treatment may be necessary. In the interest of better dental health would you then have your child take this card to a dentist of your choice. When the examination and treatment are completed, the card should be returned to school.

PRINCIPAL

FRONT

REPORT OF DENTAL EXAMINATION

This is to certify that I have examined the teeth of

--- and:

☐ 1. All necessary dental work has been completed.

☐ 2. Treatment is in progress.

☐ 3. No dental work is necessary.

Further recommendations -

- - - - - - - - - - - - - - - - -   -
DATE

P L E A S E   R E T U R N   T H I S   C A R D   T O   T H E   T E A C H E R

BACK

Fig. 10.—Standard form of dental inspection report to parents with reverse side used as a certificate of dental work completed. This form is used when there is no dental inspection in school.

encouraged to state what he knows about the child's dental health condition; how the teeth are cared for at home; and what the child's food preferences are. From this conversation, the counselor gains insight into the parent's attitudes toward dental health. This technique also permits the parent to state the problem *as he sees it.*

The counselor then presents the findings of the dental health inspection, helping the parent to gather information and understanding about dental defects and why they must be corrected. The counselor should encourage questions and answer them frankly. The parent should be encouraged to figure out possible ways of obtaining the needed dental treatment and sources that may be unknown to him may be suggested. The counselor should then try to obtain a commitment from the parent about getting the needed care. The counselor should conclude the interview as soon as possible without seeming to hurry the parent. Prolonged visits are tiresome and unproductive.

Motivation through Home Visits

A home visit is frequently necessary when parents are employed or when preschool children prevent the mother from going to the school for a conference. A home visit should be an opportunity to inform the parent about the dental health program in the school rather than to reprimand her.

The dental health educator should appreciate the role of the parents, realizing that most are doing their best in terms of their insight, their motivation and their aspirations. The parents should feel that the dental health educator, the teacher and all concerned with the child in school are working for the child's welfare; that the reason for the home visit is to develop a working relationship. A simple explanation of what is expected, *i.e.,* teeth brushed after eating, regular visits to the family dentist, etc., brings far better results in parent cooperation than a demand about "why Johnnie has not been to the dentist."

The home visit is a good time to present reading material that has been prepared for parents and to discuss the results of the school dental inspection. A home visit should be scheduled in advance in order to give the mother ample opportunity to be prepared for it. It should not be hurried, but only the time needed to inform the parent properly should be spent in the home. Too often home calls are a last resort. Ideally, they should be used as devices for giving information before emergency treatment is needed. Stress *prevention* as the keynote to dental health and see the parent before the child's dental condition becomes a problem.

How home visits increased the number of defects that were corrected is reported in a program called School Health Additional Referral Program (SHARP) instituted in School District 1 in Philadelphia, Pennsylvania, where the lowest rate for correction of physical defects prevailed. Low income and meager educational background among the predominantly Negro population made this a problem area. Dental decay was the major health problem. Community resources were available for correction of defects but were not being used by those most in need of the service. The purpose of the program was to motivate parents into *initiating action* for correction of defects in their children through effective utilization of community resources. The project was carried out by the district nurses with the cooperation of all school personnel. The nurses made daytime visits to families in which the mothers were at home. Working parents were contacted by phone.

Results: Throughout the district, 30% of children with health defects had corrections in the year preceding the initiation of the SHARP program. During the first year of the program 54% and in the second year 63% of the defects were corrected. The conclusions state that in poverty areas the rate of corrections of school children's health defects can be significantly improved by intensive health counseling of parents. The one-to-one basis of health guidance between parent and health worker establishes better rapport between school and home. Treatment is secured earlier when the parents understand the need. Smaller case loads for health personnel enable them to be more effective in motivating parents to initiate health care for their children.*

Task Force on Medicaid Supports Dental Care for Children

Appointed by the Department of Health, Education and Welfare, a special Task Force on Medicaid and Related Programs has recommended an amendment to Medicaid which would make mandatory the provision of dental care for children between the ages of five through twelve. The task force also recommended that a minimum range of basic dental care services be defined which would then be required by each state. Dental care has been optional under Medicaid and states are restricted to providing dental service on an equal basis to all eligible individuals. Forty states currently include dental care in their Medicaid programs for the needy and, in

* Campbell, M. T., Garside, A. H., Frey, M. E.: "Community Needs and How They Relate to the School Health Program: SHARP— The Needed Ingredient," American Journal of Public Health, March, 1970, p. 507.

addition, twenty-three states provide dental care for the medically indigent. If young children are included in this program a great deal more dental treatment will be available on the local level.

Questions for Review and Discussion

1. The population of the United States is growing younger. It is also growing older. Explain this dichotomy of population growth.

2. Explain why a certain group of our society bears the brunt of taxation.

3. It is said that fifteen million children live in poverty. Give five primary sources which seem to contribute to this condition.

4. If the dental health in poverty areas is at a crisis, what can be done about it?

5. Define accumulated dental defects, maintenance care and incremental care.

6. Children who are given regular dental care establish certain attitudes toward dental health habits. Explain.

7. Discuss the concept of supply and demand as related to dental treatment.

8. Discuss why dental services are not used to capacity in low-income areas. What are the obligations of community agencies in this respect?

9. Dental treatment for economically deprived children often depends on establishing eligibility for aid. What can be done about eligibility in case of an emergency?

10. Release time from school for dental appointments has been discussed pro and con. What is the consensus at this time? What provisions should be made to reduce interference with school studies? What means can be employed to prevent abuses of release time?

11. What are the responsibilities of the parents for the dental health of their children? What is meant by "family-centered dental health"?

12. "Demonstrated cases of child neglect are matters for the courts." Investigate why schools are reluctant to become involved in cases involving child neglect because of bad dental health.

13. Name the steps to be taken in counseling parents.

14. Read and report to class the conclusion of the article, "Denver's Preventive Health Program for School-Age Children" (See Selected Readings.)

15. "A toothache should never be treated in school." Give the rationale for this statement.

Selected Readings

"ADA Urges Medicaid Amendment to Permit Children's Dental Care," Journal American Dental Association, December, 1969, p. 1335.

Cowen, D. L.: "Denver's Preventive Health Program for School-Age Children," American Journal of Public Health, March, 1970, p. 515.

Frankel, J. M.: "The Child, An Incremental Program," Journal of American College of Dentists, December, 1961.

Hennon, D. K., Stookey, G. K., Muhler, J. C.: "Prevalence and Distribution of Dental Caries in Preschool Children," Journal American Dental Association, December, 1969, p. 1405.

"Principles and Criteria for Determining Medical Indigency," Report of Committee, National Council on Aging, American Journal of Public Health, October, 1964, p. 1746.

Young, W. O., Striffler, D. F.: THE DENTIST, HIS PRACTICE AND HIS COMMUNITY. W. B. Saunders Co., Philadelphia, 1964, p. 180.

THE WHITE HOUSE

WASHINGTON

February 2, 1969

Water fluoridation, a highly effective method for the prevention of tooth decay, today reaches more than 82 million Americans. Those children fortunate enough to have fluoride protection suffer less than half as much tooth decay as those who are denied it. With this in mind, it is well that we now reaffirm our goal of opening for all our children a ready access both to preventive measures such as fluoridation, and to a full regimen of personal dental care. I know that all of my fellow Americans join me in this commitment and in the task of carrying it through.

Richard Nixon

FIG. 11

Chapter 7

Preventive Measures for Dental Health

The realization that prevention and control of dental disease depend largely on patient and dentist interaction does not rule out the role of the community and the school in promoting better methods of prevention through mass education, research and political cooperation. Research with combined human and animal studies is the keynote in finding new ways of preventing dental disease and acquiring better understanding of the etiology of dental caries. Much research in the field of dental caries prevention has centered around the development and testing of fluoride and other chemical preparations applied systemically or topically to reduce caries susceptibility.

Fluorides in Drinking Water

The addition of one part per million (1ppm) of fluoride to communal water supplies has proved to be an effective method of mass control of dental caries. Experimentation has been in progress for twenty-five years and after rigorous testing and evaluation, water fluoridation is now established as an accepted procedure by most influential organizations in the health professions as safe, effective and practical.

The chemical action of fluorine during and after tooth development is not fully understood. The manner in which fluorides reduce the incidence of caries susceptibility is thought to be as follows:

1. Fluorides combine with the inorganic portion of the tooth enamel, thus rendering it less soluble in the organic acids produced in the mouth.

2. Fluorides inhibit specific bacterial action which forms the acids.

3. The effect of fluoridated water is thought to continue as long as it is used.

4. Teeth benefit most from water fluoridation during their period of development.

5. There is some evidence that the decay rate increases if children who have used fluoridated water in their early years are deprived of it in subsequent years.

About one in every three children in the United States benefits from fluoridated water. More than 70% of the population is drinking fluoridated water. The current situation in other countries is spotty. Relatively good progress is being made in the Netherlands, Czechoslovakia and the United Kingdom. Hong Kong and Singapore in the Pacific have fluoridated their water supplies and progress is good in Australia, Malaysia and New Zealand. The Assembly of the World Health Organization endorsed water fluoridation in 1969.

The resolution called on all W.H.O. members to introduce "where practicable" fluoridation of community water supplies in areas where fluoride intake is below optimal levels. Proposed by Great Britain and co-sponsored by thirty-six other delegations including those of the United States and the Soviet Union, the resolution pointed out that studies in several countries consistently show that the prevalence of dental caries is definitely low when optimal concentration of fluorides occurs naturally in water supplies. The resolution also emphasized that the adjustment of the fluoride content of water supplies to an optimal level is a practical, safe and efficient public health measure; and that scientific literature on the subject has revealed no evidence of any ill effects on health from its use. W.H.O.'s endorsement of water fluoridation will serve to encourage those nations with a high decay rate and limited dental manpower to institute fluoridation.

Antifluoridation Action

The opponents of fluoridation act collectively and use fear and doubt as a means of influencing the public to vote against fluoridation of communal water supplies. The alleged bad effects claimed range in seriousness from cancer to baldness, and include brain lesions, apathy, servility, sterility, etc., etc. After twenty-five years it is clear that the antifluoridationist leaders with their illusions will not go away although none of their claims have been substantiated. In fact, a recent article in the Kansas State Department of Health publication, *Community Health*, reports that fluoridation is a boon to aging:

> The time may not be far off when there will be good evidence to indicate that the older person may have more to gain than the child. Not only will he have better teeth (his own) and thus be able to secure better nutrition in his old age, but he may also have stronger bones, less osteoporosis and he will be less likely to fracture should he have an accidental fall.

A recent study made by a team of Harvard University physicians in northwestern North Dakota revealed that in *low-fluoride areas* twice as many women had decreased bone density and two to six times as many showed collapsed vertebrae as women in *high-fluoride* areas. A striking difference between men in high- and low-fluoride areas was in the number of calcified aortas. Men living in the high-fluoride area had

40% fewer calcified aortas. Women showed the same trend.

Although 70% of the people favor fluoridation, no favorable community action has resulted. A minority, the antifluoridationists, has delayed progress in this effort to control mass dental caries. Dr. John W. Knutson, professor of preventive dentistry and public health at the University of California Medical Center in Los Angeles, suggests: "Starting fluoridation in any community must be preceded by a decision made *directly* [our italics] by popular vote or *indirectly* [our italics] by public officials at some level of government. It is an issue that is dependent on the demands and priorities for the expenditure of public funds."[*] Therefore, it should be a politically oriented effort, and even though adverse actions have been taken by community referendums, the answer, as Dr. Knutson put it, is "not to take fluoridation out of politics, but rather to have the issue decided by city councils or administrative officials rather than by referendum."[†] According to him, at this time, "only one nation, the Republic of Ireland, has made water fluoridation compulsory. In the United States, seven states—Connecticut, Minnesota, Illinois, Delaware, Michigan, South Dakota, and Ohio—have enacted legislation to require fluoridation of public water supplies."[‡]

Dr. Knutson thinks that the role of the dentists and the dental hygienists is not that of being expert on the subject of fluoridation, but rather that of influencing political public administrators. If the cause of fluoridation of water is to win, dental personnel should frankly accept the fact that they are more than simply educating the public and the politicians. They must admit that they are propagandizing, which is definitely a political strategy. The public

[*] Knutson, J. W.: "Water Fluoridation After 25 Years," Journal American Dental Association, April, 1970, p. 767.
[†] Knutson, *Ibid.*, p. 768.
[‡] Knutson, *Ibid.*, p. 768.

must not only be informed but also they should be committed to action.

Economic Benefits of Fluoridation of Water Supplies

A six-year study designed to compare time and cost factors involved in providing regular dental care to children in fluoridated and nonfluoridated areas indicates the advantages of a public health caries prevention procedure. A detailed comparison shows the extent of economic benefits and improved dental health.

The study was conducted in fluoridated Newburgh, New York and fluoride-deficient Kingston, New York, just across the Hudson River. Periodic dental care for children during the six-year period started when the children were five and six years old. The cost of corrective dental care for children with lifelong exposure to fluoridated water is less than half of the cost for children in the nonfluoridated area. The cost of incremental care is about one-half. As a result of regular incremental care in both cities there was no need to extract any permanent teeth. The chair time required to provide examination, prophylaxis and *corrective care* was about one and one-half times more in the nonfluoridated area than in the fluoridated area. The study adds a new dimension to the benefits of water fluoridation.*

Other Benefits of Fluoridation of Communal Water Supplies

Children brought up on fluoridated water have only a third as many cavities as youngsters without this advantage. Their teeth are stronger, more attractive, and as adults, they postpone or avoid entirely the use of dentures. Their dental bills are smaller, both in childhood and in later years. Fluoridation can be adopted without

* Ast, D. B., Cons, N. C., Pollard, S. T., Garfinkel, J.: "Time and Cost Factors to Provide Regular, Periodic Dental Care for Children in Fluoridated and Non-fluoridated Areas," Journal American Dental Association, April, 1970, p. 770.

danger to the health of any child or adult. The cost of fluoridation is low compared to the benefits derived.

A Note of Caution: The artificial fluoridation of drinking water is not a cure-all. It will not protect children completely from dental decay, but it is a tremendous step forward in the control of dental caries. At the present time, it offers the best solution for population-wide application to control dental caries.

Topical Application of Fluorides in Preventive Programs

A number of clinical studies has been conducted during the past twenty-five years since the public health teams of dentists and dental hygienists under Knutson set up procedures and demonstration programs in several states to show the efficacy of topical application of sodium fluoride to the teeth of school children for the prevention of tooth decay. These investigations have led to the development of various topical fluoride procedures.

Sodium Fluoride. The recommended treatment technique for the application of 2% sodium fluoride solution is:

1. The clinical crowns of the teeth are cleaned with a standard prophylactic paste in a motor-driven rubber cup.

2. One-half of the mouth (right upper quadrant and right lower quadrant) is isolated with cotton rolls and thoroughly dried with compressed air.

3. Sodium fluoride solution is applied to the teeth with cotton applicators so that all surfaces are visibly wet. The solution is permitted to dry for three minutes. The procedure is then repeated on the left half of the mouth.

4. A series of four treatments are given at one-week intervals at the ages of 3, 7, 11, and 13.

About 40% reduction in new carious teeth has been obtained over a period of years during investigations. The advantages of sodium fluoride treatment are as follows: A multiple-chair technique (several children treated at one time) can be used by each operator; the treatments need to be repeated only four times during childhood; the solution is stable if kept in a plastic container; the taste is well accepted by children; there is no discoloration of the teeth and no irritation of soft tissues. The method lends itself well to public health procedures but cost and lack of sufficient professional personnel to make the applications have been important hindrances to a wide application of the procedure so far.

Stannous Fluoride. Mercer and Muhler are credited with perfecting the technique for applying an 8% solution of stannous fluoride. A number of investigations has shown their method to be effective in reducing dental decay.

1. A thorough prophylaxis is given. Each tooth surface is cleaned and polished with pumice for five to ten seconds. Pumice is carried between the teeth with unwaxed dental floss and the proximal surfaces of the teeth are stripped.

2. Teeth are isolated with cotton rolls and dried with compressed air. Either a quadrant or one half of the mouth can be treated at one time.

3. A freshly prepared solution is applied continually to the teeth with a cotton applicator so that teeth are kept moist with the solution for four minutes. Reapplication is required every fifteen to thirty seconds.

4. For highly susceptible children the application should be repeated every six months; for less susceptible children one application per year is recommended. Studies give conflicting results, with a range of 47% to 78% fewer new DMF surfaces among treated children.

The disadvantages of stannous fluoride are that the solution is unstable and must be made fresh for each patient. It is quite astringent and disagreeable to taste; its application is therefore unpleasant. Flavoring agents are contraindicated. The solution occasionally causes a tissue irritation manifested by gingival blanching. Pig-

mentation of teeth has been reported as a light brown color which tends to mask lesions on radiographs.

Acidulated Phosphate-fluoride. This is a relatively new agent for caries reduction. The solution contains 1.23% fluoride. The preferred procedure for application is the same as that for stannous fluoride except that the solution is stable when kept in a plastic container and a new solution need not be made for each patient.

Initial clinical studies indicate that it might possess anticariogenic properties surpassing other fluoride solutions now in use. At the end of a two-year study during which the solution was applied on an annual basis, children in a test group demonstrated a 67% reduction in DMF teeth and a 70% reduction in DMF surfaces. Other studies show less glowing statistics.

Acidulated phosphate-fluoride is reported to have none of the disadvantages of sodium or stannous fluoride. Single annual application seems sufficient. Additional investigations should be made with the acidulated phosphate-fluoride gel to compare its efficacy with that of the solution.

Stannous Hexafluorozirconate (snZrF$_6$). A 16% solution of stannous hexafluorozirconate applied on a semiannual basis showed a reduction in new DMF surfaces of 96% after 9 months. A 24% solution showed 76% less DMF surfaces after 12 months. The research is not conclusive, however, and more studies should be made.

Toxic reactions after the use of stannous hexafluorozirconate in a prophylactic paste have been reported. However, the Food and Drug Administration has requested that no further studies be initiated until adequate preclinical studies demonstrate that the compound is safe for use by people.

Fluoride Prophylactic Pastes

A dental prophylaxis is prescribed to precede the application of any of the fluoride preparations. It is therefore evident that if the fluoride could be incorporated into the prophylactic paste, two operations could be consolidated into one. Bibby evaluated a paste containing 1% sodium fluoride in 1946 and reported 25% to 43% reduction in DMF teeth, depending on the number of treatments given. The United States Air Force and the University of Indiana have both developed a stannous fluoride prophylactic paste. A silex silicone base was used for the paste. It was found to be seriously lacking as a material for cleaning and polishing teeth.

The aqueous stannous fluoride-lava pumice prophylactic paste tasted better, cleaned better and was less irritating to the gingiva than the silex silicone paste. An average reduction of 34% in DMF teeth was noted for the pumice paste at the end of one year. When it was followed by the application of 8% stannous fluoride treatment the gain was still greater. Results after two or three years showed that the agents continued to maintain their effectiveness. Further study is needed to confirm the efficiency of any of the fluoride-containing prophylactic pastes. Conflicting findings place the efficacy of these agents in doubt.

Self-administration of Topical Fluorides

The increasing shortage of manpower and the relatively high cost of treatment accentuate the shortcomings of a professionally administered technique as a public health measure. Research projects are in progress to discover whether self-applied prophylactic pastes brushed on the teeth at stated intervals will reduce the DMF rate. Published data strongly suggest that the self-administration of topical fluorides may provide an answer to the problems of insufficient professional manpower and excessive costs that hinder topical fluoride programs. Self-administration will probably become the method of choice when improvements are made in therapeutic agents and when techniques for self-application are improved. At this time, there is insuf-ficient evidence to recommend any self-administration procedure, be it with tooth-brushing, mouth rinses or mouth pieces for general use in public health programs.

Topical Fluoride Application in Optimum Fluoride Areas

The American Dental Association recommends that "in those communities which undertake water fluoridation, the topical application of fluorides should be continued for those children whose teeth were calcified or erupted at the time fluoridation was initiated." Because the effectiveness of topical fluorides in areas where children have received the full benefits of water fluoridation has not been sufficiently documented, the procedure cannot be currently recommended for public health programs in those areas.*

Fluoride Tablets for Children

There are situations in which some other way of adding fluorides to the diet would be more effective and convenient. Various methods have been suggested from time to time. A study made in 1960 by the National Institute of Dental Health proved a method of individual supervision by a dentist effective. A sodium fluoride tablet (1.0 mg) was dissolved in regulated quantities of water, milk or fruit juice according to the child's age and given at stated intervals.

There has been little or no use of this method except in dental practice where individual children who have high susceptibility to dental caries can be carefully supervised. The use of fluoride tablets should be considered a prescription medication to be used under the direction of a dentist only. Mass medication of this type is not recommended because the effects on individuals can not be controlled.

* Adapted from "Council on Dental Therapeutics, Accepted Dental Therapeutics, 1969-1970." American Dental Association, Chicago, 1969, p. 193.

Prevention through Adequate Nutrition

This subject has been treated at some length in Chapter 2. Nutrition is the sum of the processes by which the body takes in and utilizes food. It includes diet, digestion and metabolism. The individual and family diet over a long period of time becomes established by habit; it is difficult to change. The main concern of dental health instruction is to show the relationship between good general health and an adequate diet; to try to influence children and adults to eat the four basic foods in recommended quantities every day; and to stress the quality and characteristics of foods that have a direct bearing on good mouth hygiene.

The harmful effects of sugars left on the teeth, particularly by eating snacks high in sugar content, should be stressed.

Improved Mouth Hygiene Schedules

A number of studies supports the evidence that effective brushing of the teeth improves gingival health, retards the formation of calculus and plaque and reduces the number of cavities. The onset of periodontal disease is arrested by good toothbrushing and a full regime of mouth care.

There has been a noticeable change in the period of time recommended for toothbrushing. Morning and night brushing is not considered sufficient for good mouth hygiene. Brushing after eating, including snacks, is advised for the reduction of food debris and the prevention of acid formation. It requires a complete change in the toothbrushing routine in some households. The effectiveness of oral hygiene procedures is more a matter of technique, effort and timing than the materials used as dentifrices and mouthwashes. The condition of the toothbrush, new or old and soft, is more important than the brand used. The size and shape that fits the individual mouth is important as well as the texture of the brush. Recommendations of the dentist are the best guide to selecting brushes, dentifrices and mouthwashes. The method of brushing is also one that should meet the need of each individual mouth. Children are usually taught the American Dental Association method of brushing. Adults are advised to brush for three minutes. Children brush ten strokes in each area of the mouth.

A number of electric toothbrushes have been tested and found to be efficient if supervised instruction is provided. Brushes that have a short reciprocal stroke and a strong motor are more effective than other types. Adolescents react favorably to using electric toothbrushes. The mechanical element appeals to them.

The use of a pulsating water jet device can reduce gingival debris after toothbrushing, but the effect on calculus and plaque is questionable. Water jets should not be used in place of good, vigorous toothbrushing.

The use of wood picks for gingival stimulation is recommended for patients in whom periodontal involvement is apparent. It is not advised for patients with healthy teeth with normal gingival attachment which may be injured by too strenuous use. Unwaxed dental floss and tape for cleaning plaque and debris from areas that are otherwise missed are recommended. Vigorous rinsing after brushing is an excellent means of removing food debris but does not take the place of toothbrushing.

A motivating device that is effective is use of disclosing solution or tablets. The tablets are chewed, the mouth is rinsed and the red coloring adheres to the plaque and calculus missed by toothbrushing. Painting disclosing solutions on teeth is a part of the professional prophylactic treatment. When they are used before and after brushing, the tablets show places that are missed by the brush. Checking the efficiency of toothbrushing tends to make it important to the patient and to keep his interest in a clean mouth.

The Effect of Dental Health Education in Preventive Dental Hygiene

A set routine in mouth hygiene which becomes an unconscious habit is a good health asset. Mouth health saves money, cuts short visits to the dentist, improves appearance and increases self-esteem and morale. Dental health instruction leads to increased knowledge and a greater interest in maintaining mouth health. The quality, timing and intensity of the instruction have a decided effect on the motivation of the individual. This subject will be treated more in detail in the next section of the text.

Questions for Review and Discussion

1. Discuss why the issue of fluoridating a communal water supply is a political one. How is it best solved?

2. What can be done to combat the effects of antifluoridationists?

3. "Regular and adequate dental treatment is the only *sure* method of controlling dental caries." In light of all the other preventive measures that have received approval by organized dentistry, why is this statement still true?

4. Name the several chemical compounds of fluorine that have received approval as topically applied preventive measure for the control of dental caries.

5. What are the disadvantages of the *mass* application of fluorides to tooth surfaces as they relate to public health programs?

6. It is said that in the future mass application of topical fluorides will be possible and expedient by *self-application.* Discuss this statement.

7. What is the effect of topically applied fluorides on children who have had the full advantages of living in fluoridated areas?

8. What is the status of the several fluoride-containing prophylactic pastes?

9. Certain fluoridated toothpastes have been "accepted by the American Dental Association." How is this acceptance obtained (research question)?

10. State your philosophy on the role of dental health education in a preventive dental health program.

Selected Readings

"A Guide to Reading on Fluoridation," Public Health Service Publication No. 1680, U.S. Public Health Service, Dental Division, 8120 Woodmont Ave., Bethesda, Md. 20014.

Gravelle, H. R., Schackelford, M. F., Lovett, J. T.: "The Oral Hygiene of High School Students as Affected by Three Different Educational Programs." Journal Public Health Dentistry, Spring, 1967, p. 91.

Hoover, D. R., Robinson, H. B. G.: "The Comparative Effectiveness of the Water-Pik in a Noninstructed Population," Journal Periodontology, January, 1968, p. 47.

Horowitz, H.: "Call for Fluoridation of School Water Supplies," Journal American Dental Association, Annual Sessions Bulletin, November, 1969.

Knutson, J. W.: "Water Fluoridation After 25 Years," Journal American Dental Association, April, 1970, p. 765.

Lobene, R. R., Soparker, P. M.: "Effect of a Pulsed Water Pressure Cleansing Device on Oral Health," IADR Abstract No. 344, 1969.

"Prentive Dentistry," film and pamphlet, Patient Counseling Film Program, American Dental Association, 1969.

Ritsert, E. F., Binns, W. H.: "Adolescents Brush Better with an Electric Toothbrush," Journal of Dentistry for Children, September, 1967, p. 354.

Sims, W.: "Interpretation and Use of Synder Tests and Lactobacillus Counts," Journal American Dental Association, June, 1970, p. 1315.

Sumnicht, R. W.: "Research in Preventive Dentistry," Journal American Dental Association, November, 1969, p. 1193.

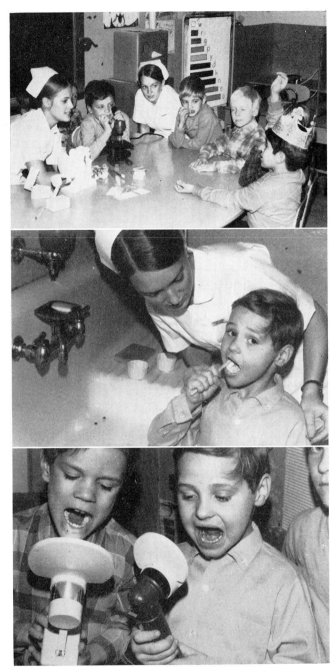

FIG. 12.—As part of a research project, dental hygienists teach dental health to exceptional (i.e., of low mentality) children in small groups. Each child is taught to brush his teeth and practices under supervision of the dental hygienist. The children view in illuminated mirrors the results of their toothbrushing efforts. (Courtesy, Department of Dental Hygiene, School of Dentistry, University of Minnesota.)

Chapter 8

The Community Dental Health Program

The prevention and control of disabilities, whether physical, mental or emotional, are most effective when efforts start early in life. Health education begins with birth and should continue through the entire span of life—in the home, in the school and in the community. Because preventive hygiene for the *prevention* of disease and personal hygiene for the *promotion* of positive health are based upon the application of health knowledge by the individual, organized dental health education has become an important factor in public health programs.

Any goal to improve health should have a common purpose that gives unity and direction to all efforts. In the case of dental health, it is to provide the opportunity for everyone to maintain a sound complement of teeth in a healthy mouth for a lifetime.

The solutions to the numerous problems of dental health described in the previous chapters can be achieved through careful planning based on accurate knowledge of the extent of dental disease; the degree of severity to which the disease has progressed; the means available for alleviating the disease; and the potential resources for preventing and controlling further development of dental disabilities. The local community is unique in its dental health problems. The solutions to these problems will be found at the local level. Progress can be made by community action so that all citizens will have a reasonable opportunity for dental health.

Dental Health in the Family

Parents have the duty and responsibility for giving guidance to children in establishing good dental health habits and practices in the home. Children need to know long before they enter school that brushing the teeth after each meal and after between-meal snacks is the rule of the home. Parents must teach children to avoid accidents. Falls are responsible for nearly half of the home accidents. Many of these affect the front teeth. Most parents seek medical care for an injured child, but few parents consider injuries to the teeth of small children serious, yet premature loss of primary teeth leads to malocclusion, and at times, loss of permanent teeth.

Regular dental treatment started at the age of three years should be provided for in every family budget. These services will usually be given by the family dentist. Many dental disabilities begin early in life, and if they are recognized at one of the periodical visits, can be prevented. Parents cannot depend on their own observation to determine accurately a child's needs. Early and regular visits to the family dentist are the obligation of every parent for every child. The community should provide dental health services, and instruction for those parents who are unable to provide treatment for their children.

Children need at least three wholesome meals each day, served in a congenial family atmosphere. A good diet supplies

71

Table 2. *The Community Dental Health Program*

* Official Agency Dental Program	† Voluntary Agency Dental Program	School Dental Health Program	Dental Association Program	Home Dental Health Program
Research	Treatment clinics	Dental inspections	Stimulus for school and community programs	Establishes good dental health practices
Surveys and analyses	Financial support	Graded instruction	Speakers	
Public relations	Aid to indigents	Counseling	Authentic information	Adequate dental treatment for each child
Speakers	Educational materials	Follow-up	Financial aid	
Printed information	Funds for dental treatment	Referral for treatment	Professional guidance	Wholesome food in congenial atmosphere
Parent education		Parent participation	Dental treatment for the population	
Community resources		Remedial services	Professional personnel	Informed on dental health facts
Coordination of existing programs				
				Participation in dental health efforts of school and community

* National, state, and local (county, city, town). Publicly financed.
† Foundations, philanthropic organizations, semiofficial agencies, service clubs. Privately financed.

substances the body needs for growth and repair. Children learn eating habits at home that remain with them for life. It is during these formative years that the restriction of free sugars which are the main cause of tooth decay can be learned. American children consume more sugar than any other children in the world. They are fed sweet food in their earliest bottle feeding. All children need energy foods but these should be restricted in quantity and should be eaten at the end of the meal, not as snacks. Lunches packed at home should contain some detergent food such as an apple, celery, carrot or other raw fruit or vegetable to remove food remaining on the teeth when brushing is not possible.

Parents should be well informed in dental health facts and willing to act accordingly. Every community has some resources which are frequently unknown and unused by those who need help. Parents are often unable to provide the necessary dental treatment for a number of reasons. Parents should be encouraged to consult the dental health personnel of the school and the community agencies with the assurance that their children will not be known as "charity cases."

The Role of Voluntary Agencies in Dental Health Education

Voluntary health agencies are those groups of people who are interested in furthering the health status of the community through independent action. They usually work with official government agencies. They may establish and support dental health clinics for indigent children or provide funds for the treatment of children under a fee-for-service plan. They provide volunteer services for clerical tasks in health agencies, for transporting children to dental appointments, for raising funds and for distributing dental health literature prepared by professional dental health educators. They are frequently responsible for bringing dental health problems of the community to the attention of officials and citizens so that action may result.

These organizations often join together in community health councils in order to coordinate their services and to prevent overlapping of effort. Any group formed in the community for the purpose of furthering better dental health should be a cross section of the community population. It should include representative citizens from the medical and dental professions but should not be led or dominated by those who have vested interests in either medicine or dentistry.

Responsibilities of Community Agencies for Dental Health

Community agencies, official and voluntary, have a number of definite purposes and responsibilities for the dental health of the community. They are as follows:

A. Survey and Interpret Dental Status of the Population. If the schools in small communities do not have funds to employ dental health personnel to carry on a full-scale dental health education program, public health agencies on the local or county level may assume this responsibility by providing dental inspections in order to determine the needs of the community.

B. Appraise the Dental Health Needs of the Community. Estimates of the needs of the community as to treatment resources for the dental care of children are obtained by analyzing the data collected. Is it necessary to establishing clinical services to augment the present services rendered by the local dentists in order to provide for the needs of underprivileged children? Should these facilities be financed through tax funds or would some other form of financing such as a small fee-for-service provide funds for staffing the clinic? These and many other questions are best solved through public health agencies working with the local voluntary agencies.

C. Provide Authentic Dental Health Information. The official and voluntary agencies provide information through trained dental health personnel. Authentic printed materials are distributed to parents and children. The Bureau of Dental Health of the American Dental Association will provide quantities of materials on dental health for a small fee. A number of commercial companies contribute sums of money for producing informational materials. Some companies provide excellent materials to be distributed by community agencies and local dentists.

D. *Organize Community Efforts to Improve Dental Health.* Americans are community-minded people. When they recognize a problem, they are usually eager to find ways and means of solving it. Dental health is recognized as a community problem and many efforts are made to solve it. Each community, with the aid of public health agencies, attempts to solve its problem through community health councils. It offers special inducements to increase the number of local dentists to alleviate dental manpower shortages and organizes treatment centers. Preschool round-up for young children that includes dental inspections and parental instruction in good dental health procedures is usually conducted by schools with the aid of voluntary community agencies. These are but a few of the efforts made to solve problems of dental health on the community level.

E. *Provide Funds for Community Dental Projects.* Service clubs provide much of the financial aid needed to carry out dental health projects. Money may be provided to individual families who can then choose their own dentists, thus keeping freedom of choice within the family. Local banks provide loans for dental treatment. Local philanthropies finance clinics which are operated by the volunteer services of the local dental and dental hygienist associations. Generalized funds such as community chests allocate a percentage of their funds to dental health programs.

F. *Coordinate Various Phases of Community Dental Health Efforts.* In an or-

ganized democratic society it is necessary to eliminate duplication of effort so that the most benefit for the greatest number of people will be obtained for money spent. The community health council can produce excellent results by bringing together representatives of local agencies to exchange information so that the objectives and purposes of each group in reference to the whole community effort are clarified and duplication reduced.

G. *Evaluate Community Efforts.* Unless periodic review of what is being done in community projects is made, deterioration of effort due to lack of stimulus is likely. Official and voluntary agencies offer professional guidance in appraising progress. The local dental society provides a true assessment of the local dental health status. Who knows the community problems better than the professional men who work directly with the people of the community? Constant evaluation stimulates interest and clarifies objectives. Since dental health is a continuous challenge with many unsolved facets, evaluation becomes a necessary part of any community effort. Are we traveling in the right direction? Are there better ways of doing what we have continued to do for several years? Answers are found through evaluating efforts.

H. *Provide and Publish Periodic Reports on Community Progress.* This item is a corollary to evaluation. It provides the public with tangible evidence that something is being done about a problem. Reports also show the need for further effort by indicating inadequacies that exist and suggesting possible additional means of meeting these needs. Reports not only provide information; they also become a means of stimulating public interest.

I. *Organize and Maintain Treatment Services and Guidance for Indigents.* The care of indigents rightfully belongs to the official agencies of the government. However, voluntary agencies have led the way by organizing services for the needy, thus indicating to the official agencies that need exists. After the need has been demonstrated and the official agency takes over management of the problem, voluntary agencies tend to relinquish their efforts and to turn attention to another area of need. Many of our public welfare programs originated in actions by voluntary agencies.

J. Stimulate Community Action by Support of Legislation and Other Efforts for Better Dental Health. Professional organizations composed of teachers, nurses, physicians, dentists and dental hygienists have one or more standing committees that have the responsibility of watching proposed bills that may affect the welfare of their associations. They support those bills which will help the population at large and oppose those that tend to favor pressure groups. Through their congressmen they may initiate bills that are designed to solve community health problems. In recent years many states have passed bills authorizing the addition of fluorides to water supplies. This action can be traced directly to the organized efforts of dental and dental hygienist associations.

The Community Health Council

The community health council is shown in figure 13. It is essentially a technique for planning and carrying out projects wisely and with a minimum of wasted time and resources. The health council was developed to meet local needs for a coordinating and voluntary body of representative public-spirited citizens. The purpose of the council is primarily to promote and support public and private health efforts; to serve as a forum for discussion of problems, policies and plans; to improve standards of service; to secure improvement in existing facilities; to suggest new health

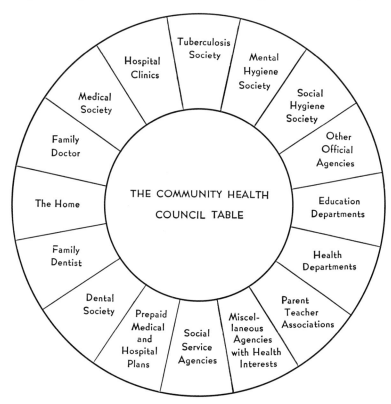

Fig. 13.—The community health council table. Coordinate representation—no loss of identity—separate administration—voluntary cooperation—duplication eliminated—efficiency enhanced. (Reproduced from Health Education, courtesy, National Education Association.)

services; to indicate duplication of effort; and to give moral support to official programs in cooperation with the professional and official organizations.

The School Dental Health Program as It Relates to Public Health

All states have some provision in the education laws for medical examinations. The laws vary widely in the type and extent of examinations, but they all require that some type of instruction in health topics be included in the curriculum. The present program of health activities in public schools has evolved gradually from the early days of public education when the school was concerned with little beyond teaching of purely factual information.

About 1880 every state had passed a law requiring instruction concerning the ill effects of alcohol and tobacco. In 1903 the first dentist was employed to do dental examinations in the schools of Reading, Pennsylvania, and in 1914 ten dental hygienists were introduced into the schools of Bridgeport, Connecticut for the purpose of cleaning the teeth of all the children as a means of preventing dental decay. Dental health instruction was included in the classrooms and during prophylaxis. The dental hygienists were recognized as special educators in dental health. The practice of employing dental hygienists in school health plans has spread widely throughout the United States.

During 1918 and the years following World War I there was a widespread interest in the promotion of health through health education in schools which was stimulated by the number of draftees who were rejected by the armed forces because of physical disabilities. Today there is another upsurge of interest in health instruction programs because of the use of narcotics and hallucinogenic drugs. The tendency toward sexual experimentation among teen-agers has sent up a cry for better family life education in the upper elementary grades and high school. Dental

health instruction continues to receive increasing support as parents realize the need for early regular dental care based on good dental health information.

Present-day responsibilities for health in schools deal with: 1. health protection; 2. the correction of defects; and 3. health promotion by building good health concepts based on authentic information and motivating the individual to practice good health routines. These topics will be covered in depth in Part III of the text.

The Role of the Dental Hygienist in Public Health Programs

The role of the dental hygienist in public health and school dental health programs is being given added importance as the dental health programs in state and local levels increase. The dental hygienist is required to have the same essential background of education that is required of other health personnel of equal rank— knowledge and skill in public health and education procedures as well as the basic professional training and licensure.

The Committee on Professional Education of the American Public Health Association approved a statement of the functions of the dental hygienist in public health. These are as follows:

1. Provide dental prophylaxis and other oral hygiene measures, including instruction in home care of the mouth.

2. Apply caries preventive measures such as topical applications of fluorides.

3. Demonstrate new dental preventive methods and procedures to other dental hygienists and allied health workers.

4. Participate as a dental health adviser in community health activities such as well child conferences, expectant parent classes, prenatal conferences and readiness for school programs.

5. Assist in community dental surveys, including the inspection, recording, analysis and interpretation of the data to the community.

6. Assist a community in planning, or-

ganizing and conducting a dental health program suitable to the needs and resources of the area.

7. Assist in planning and conducting preservice and inservice training programs in dental health for: (*a*) other public health personnel, (*b*) school personnel and (*c*) civic groups interested in dental health.

8. Assist in planning and conducting dental public health activities and field experiences for student dental hygienists and student nurses.

9. Assist in planning and conducting school dental health programs by: (*a*) serving as a resource person in dental health to teachers, administrators and other school personnel, (*b*) performing dental inspections of children, establishing referral and follow-through systems for dental care, (*c*) maintaining records on the dental status of school children, (*d*) providing dental prophylaxis and topical fluoride treatments for school children on either a demonstration or service basis, (*e*) evaluating, developing, and making available dental health educational material to interested persons.

10. Assist voluntary health agencies, civic groups and dental or allied professional groups in carrying out special dental health activities.

The future development of dental public health programs will show that by expanding the services that dental hygienists are permitted to perform, greater services can be offered to the public. Expanded duties have been under consideration for at least twenty years. Little or no progress can be reported at this time although there is an upsurge of interest among members of the dental profession who are concerned about the shortage of dental manpower. Dentists alone cannot hope to provide all the care demanded and needed by an informed population. Most of the opposition to expanding the services dental hygienists can render comes from a limited number of dentists who fear socialization of dentistry. Efforts continue to provide the public with additional dental services by expand-

ing the field of practice of dental hygienists. The movement is supported by the American Dental Hygienists' Association and the American Dental Association.

Questions for Review and Discussion

1. The local community is unique in its dental health problems; therefore, the solutions to these problems will be found at this level. With this statement in mind, make a survey of a local neighborhood and ascertain (1) the extent of the dental health problem among school children; (2) list the resources for dental care available for indigents; (3) how many dentists have offices in the neighborhood; (4) what is the economic status of the several ethnic groups who are residents?

2. After completing the survey make recommendations on how dental health in that community can be improved.

3. Describe a good regimen of dental health to be carried out daily in the home.

4. What is meant by a wholesome diet?

5. List a number of ways that parents can become "involved" in the dental health program of the community.

6. Financial resources are always a problem in community efforts to provide dental care for indigents. Name several sources from which aid can be secured.

7. Legislative efforts frequently miscarry and provide laws that are not in the best interest of the community or the individual. How can professional people "watchdog" the numerous bills which are introduced in the legislatures?

8. Accidents to teeth are commonplace in the home. What immediate action should be taken if teeth appear to have been injured?

9. Define: official agency, voluntary agency, community health council.

Selected Readings

Breslow, L.: "The Urgency of Social Action for Health," American Journal of Public Health, January, 1970, p. 10.

Colt, A. M.: "Elements of Comprehensive Health

Planning," American Journal of Public Health, July, 1970, p. 1194.

"Introduction to Dental Public Health," U.S. Dept. Health, Education, and Welfare, Public Health Service Publication No. 1134, 1964.

Kaiser, L. R., Ver Steeg, M. A., Abell, J.: "Strategies for Effective Utilization of Underprivileged Youth in Public Health Education," American Journal of Public Health, February, 1970, p. 340.

Muller, Charlotte: "Program Elements of Federal Laws on Financing of Health Facilities,"

American Journal of Public Health, February, 1970, p. 305.

"Report from Washington," monthly articles in the Journal of American Dental Association on pending legislation and other items of interest to dentistry.

Schaefer, A. E.: "Nutrition Survey in Low-Income Areas," U.S. Public Health Service, reviewed in J.A.D.A. April, 1969, p. 723.

Young, W. O., Striffler, D. F.: THE DENTIST, HIS PRACTICE AND HIS COMMUNITY, W. B. Saunders Co., Philadelphia, 1964.

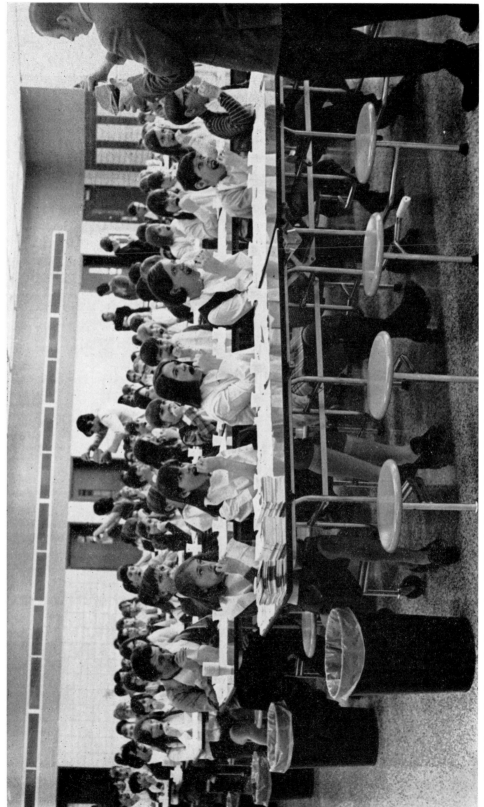

Fig. 14.—A brush-in demonstration during Children's Dental Health Week, which is promoted by the Regional Dental Hygienists with the cooperation of the local dental society, the school nurses and interested members of the community. (Courtesy, Dental Health Program, Commonwealth of Pennsylvania.)

Chapter 9

A Successful State-wide Dental Health Plan

The Commonwealth of Pennsylvania Dental Health Program

In the preceding chapters a foundation has been laid for understanding the individual and the community needs of the population for better dental health. This chapter focuses upon the application of principles in a state-wide dental health program. The dental health program of the Commonwealth of Pennsylvania, which has had an outstanding dental health program since 1920, is used as a model. It was one of the early programs to employ dental hygienists in the schools and through the years the State Department of Health, Division of Dental Hygiene has revised and changed its function to meet the changing needs of the people and the expanding economy of the state. The program represents a combined administrative structure of the State Department of Health and the Department of Education.

The state law makes dental examinations by dentists mandatory:

"*Article 322, section B.* Dental examinations on original entry into school and in the third and seventh grades. In instances where there are kindergartens in some schools of a district and not in others, the board or joint board may decide whether medical and dental examinations shall begin in the first grade or in the kindergarten.

"Dental examinations shall be done with such care and detail as to command dental respect and to provide an educational experience for the child and his parents. Examinations will be scheduled so that on an average no more than eight children will be examined in an hour. The school dental examination may be done by the family dentist and reported to the school on forms supplied by the school. Administrators are urged to have as many children examined privately as possible as this provides for continuity in the child's dental care. Payment for such examinations are the responsibility of the parent. However, children examined privately will still be counted as part of the enrollment for reimbursement purposes.

"Children transferred from other school systems shall be examined as soon as possible after the transfer regardless of their age or grade if an adequate dental record is not made available by the original school."

There was a feeling that the three examinations were not benefiting the dental health of children and this was confirmed by a state-wide survey in 1963. As a result a bill was passed in the state legislature the same year permitting school districts to have a choice of the *mandated examination* (required by law) by a dentist or a program of *dental hygiene* services conducted by public health dental hygienists and supervised by dentists. This is *permissive legislation* (allowed but not required by law) and it permits school districts to receive state funds to pay the salaries of the dental hygienists employed by them to conduct the dental hygiene service program.

The expanded state program has the basic objective of providing:

A. Consultative and supportive services
B. Demonstration projects
C. Continuing education programs for personnel
D. Local project grants

The Dental Hygiene Section of the Dental Division defines the problem as one of an education which provides factual information and through motivation develops favorable behavorial patterns. Although the effectiveness of dental health education is difficult to measure, the increase and extension of dental health education and dental hygiene services in the communities indicate progress in achieving goals.

The objectives of the dental health program are to improve existing dental health education programs in schools and to extend such health education on a broader basis throughout the community. Efforts are made to increase community acceptance of comprehensive dental hygiene services in the school programs and to extend the dental hygiene services into the community programs.

Fluoride Supplement Program

In areas where the water supply is not fluoridated, dietary fluoride tablet programs are initiated to help prevent dental caries. Currently, these programs are operating in public schools, Head Start programs, child health conferences and day care centers, special education classes, and centers for the mentally and physically handicapped child. There are 110 dietary fluoride programs operating in the public schools which are benefiting approximately 43,942 children. Preschool children receiving the fluoride supplement number approximately 1,400.

Dental health education is provided in well baby clinics and projects relating to nutrition. Dental health instruction is given in the Head Start and day care programs.

Brush-in Programs. The mass self-application of fluoride by using prophylactic pastes as a caries-reduction measure has been used in ten school districts; 4328 pupils in grades 6 to 12 participated in

ORGANIZATION PLAN 1970-1971

```
            ┌─────────────────┐
            │    COMMUNITY    │
            │     HEALTH      │
            │    PLANNING     │
            └─────────────────┘

          Continuing Education

          Interagency Relationships

            ┌─────────────────┐
            │ DIVISION DIRECTOR│
            └─────────────────┘

┌──────────────┐  ┌──────────────┐  ┌──────────────┐
│  COMMUNITY   │  │    DENTAL    │  │    DENTAL    │
│   HEALTH     │  │   HYGIENE    │  │   SERVICES   │
│   SECTION    │  │   SECTION    │  │   SECTION    │
└──────────────┘  └──────────────┘  └──────────────┘
```

Table 3. *Operational Programs*

Community Health Section	Dental Hygiene Section	Dental Services Section

Community diagnosis
Fluoridation promotion
School fluoridation
	Dental health education
	School dental hygiene services
	Topical fluoride program
	Dietary fluoride supplement
	  programs
	Mass toothbrush demonstration
	  or brush-ins
	Consultative services to health
	  and teaching personnel in
	  special schools and hospitals
		Dentofacial program

Demonstration Programs

Oral cytology
Preventive orthodontics
Periodontal disease
  prevention
	Screening
	Fluoride prophylaxis
	Dietary supplement for special
	  education classes
	Pilot schools for mentally and
	  physically handicapped
		Care of handicapped, chronically
		  ill and aged
		Survey of facilities and resources

Research—Field Studies—Special Projects

School topical fluoride
Fluoride supplements
Caries-susceptibility testing

Table 4

Primary Preventive Procedure	Objective of Procedure
Dental Caries	
a. water fluoridation b. prophylaxis c. topical fluoride d. nutrition counseling e. mouth hygiene instruction f. fluoride supplement	a. caries reduction b. removal of dental plaque c. reduction in enamel solubility d. reduction of sugar intake e. reduction of plaque formation f. caries reduction
Periodontal Disease	
a. prophylaxis b. mouth hygiene instruction	a. removal of dental plaque and calculus b. reduction of plaque and calculus formation; maintaining tone of the supporting tissues
Acquired Malocclusion	

a. all the above
b. patient counseling
	a. prevention of premature loss of teeth which
	  causes adjacent teeth to shift position
	b. prevention of habits which force teeth out
	  of position

HDH 25025 REV. 10/65

COMMONWEALTH OF PENNSYLVANIA
DEPARTMENT OF HEALTH
DENTAL HEALTH

SCHOOL DENTAL HEALTH RECORD

SCHOOL DISTRICT	COUNTY	POST OFFICE		
NAME OF STUDENT LAST FIRST MIDDLE		AGE NEAREST BIRTHDAY		
HOME ADDRESS		GRADE	SEX M ☐ F ☐	RACE W ☐ NON-W ☐

THE ABOVE INFORMATION SHOULD BE FILLED IN BEFORE THE EXAMINATION OR SCREENING

RECOMMENDATIONS FOR PREVENTIVE SERVICES (COMPLETE REFERRAL RECORD BELOW)

DATE	PROPHYLAXIS	TOPICAL F APPLICATION	TOOTHBRUSH INSTRUCTION	NUTRITION COUNSELING	SPACE MAINTAINER	REMARKS

PATIENT REFERRAL RECORD

DATE	REFERRED BY	REFERRED TO	REMARKS ON FOLLOW-UP

Fig. 15.—(*Continued on opposite page.*)

Grade	Date	DENTAL FINDINGS — Examined or Screened By	No. Years Drinking Fluoridated Water	Topical F Applications (Date)	PATIENT CLASSIFICATION -- CHECK ONE (SEE REVERSE SIDE) CLASS 1 Patient Under Care of Family Dentist	CLASS 2 School Dental Hygiene Service Patient	CLASS 3 Treatment Patient (Referral for Care)	Urgent Need?	CLASS 4 Special Problem (Specify)	Classification Changed To:
K										
1										
2										
3										
4										
5										
6										
7										
8										
9										
10										
11										
12										

NAME OF STUDENT _____

PATIENT CLASSIFICATION

CLASS 1. PATIENT UNDER CARE OF A FAMILY DENTIST.

CLASS 2. SCHOOL DENTAL HYGIENE SERVICE PATIENT (NO URGENT OR EXTENSIVE TREATMENT REQUIREMENTS, BUT HAVING NEWLY ERUPTED, SOUND PERMANENT TEETH; RECOMMENDED FOR PREVENTIVE PROGRAM.)

CLASS 3. TREATMENT PATIENT (NEEDING DENTAL CARE; REQUIRING REFERRAL TO FAMILY DENTIST OR COMMUNITY DENTAL CLINIC.)

CLASS 4. SPECIAL PROBLEM (HAVING DENTAL PROBLEM REQUIRING SPECIALIZED CARE, E. G. DENTOFACIAL DEFORMITY OR HANDICAPPING CONDITION.)

CLASSIFICATION MAY BE CHANGED DURING SCHOOL YEAR DEPENDING UPON PATIENT'S NEEDS

FIG. 15.—School Dental Health Forms—Commonwealth of Pennsylvania.

these brush-ins. A paste of 9% stannous fluoride or 2.2% sodium fluoride is recommended for use at least once a year.

Topical Fluoride Programs. The number of elementary school children who have received a topical fluoride treatment is 55,000. These treatments were either a fluoride solution, a fluoride gel or a prophylactic paste containing fluoride.

In order to attain these objectives the state regional staff will continue to provide consultant services to improve the school dental health education program by including demonstrations of the latest educational aids. Particular emphasis is placed on the school dental hygiene services, in which program planning and evaluation are offered.

Dental health services are concerned with the primary prevention of dental disease. Dental hygiene services qualify as primary preventive procedures as follows:

It is generally agreed among those in public dental health that primary preventive procedures should receive priority in dental health programs for children of school age. However, this is contrary to the thinking in educational circles, where dental health education is the primary function. The program sequence in primary preventive procedures is:

1. Dental hygiene services should take precedence over
2. Early detection of defects through oral examinations, and
3. Restoration of dental defects.

To be effective, all three procedures, essential to a comprehensive school dental program, should include appropriate follow-up measures.

Evaluation of the Program

It is expected that success of the program will be indicated by an increase in the number of schools showing improvement in the dental health programs; by an increase in the number of schools that adopt the dental hygiene service program;

by an increase in the number of community projects which use the dental hygienists' services; how many schools use the consultant services of the state regional staff; and by the increase in participation in conferences, training programs and traineeships by dental hygiene personnel.

Discussion and Conclusions

The outstanding feature of this program is the emphasis on dental health education through all its community phases. There is a clear indication that the public health team approach is used to best advantage to provide dental health services. The continuing educational program for the personnel should insure staff interest and stimulation by dentists and the dental hygienists who are designated as the primary dental health educators.*

The individual dental health record is complete and indicates that data for a number of research projects, such as the number of years of drinking fluoridated water and the number of topical fluoride applications, are being collected as part of the dental health service program in the schools. The dental health record is designed to compile information from kindergarten through high school and since it has been adopted on a state-wide basis, it is transferable from school to school, a distinct advantage to the school, the child and the continuation of the research projects.

Pennsylvania's public health dental program goes beyond the schools into the community areas of need by proposing to provide initial and incremental dental care for children and to include, for the handicapped, the chronically ill and aged, special care and hospital dental services.

There is little disagreement between educators and public health authorities upon the goals for good dental health. Both groups agree that every American child

* Personal communication from Louise Coira, R. D. H., Chief of Dental Hygiene Section, State Department of Health, Commonwealth of Pennsylvania, September 1970.

should have the right to grow up with a full complement of healthy teeth, but they differ about the means by which these goals may be reached. Educators place emphasis upon instruction as the means of motivating people to practice good dental health habits in the belief that the informed individual will find the means of obtaining good dental health through self-discipline and responsibility. On the other hand, public health personnel regard primary prevention as an obligation of the state in providing fluoridated water and topical application of fluorides as the means of obtaining good dental health for the largest group of the population. Dental inspections or examinations are considered secondary prevention rather than an educative opportunity, as it is considered by educators. Dental health education permeates the public health programs so that every opportunity to instruct individuals and groups is used to advantage. Organized curricula for dental health instruction are favored as part of the educative process in schools, with incidental teaching as an adjunct to learning and to the application of dental health facts.

Questions for Review and Discussion

1. What are the advantages of studying a complete program of dental hygiene in a state public health situation?

2. Why did the law mandate the examination of school children by dentists? What motivated the change to permit dental hygienists to inspect children's teeth?

3. Define "primary prevention" as it applies to dental health programs. Give examples of such measures.

4. What effort is made to establish caries susceptibility in individual children? Is it practical? What advantages or disadvantages are there in this procedure?

5. What are the advantages of a preschool dental service program?

6. How do the objectives of the public health program differ from a department of education program in the schools?

7. What financial advantage to school districts is implied in the amended law permitting a school dental service program?

8. What dental health services will a child receive if he is placed in Class 2 following the screening inspection?

9. What precautions have been taken to preserve the family dentist relationships?

10. How has the State Department of Health guaranteed participation in the dental hygiene program by the local dentists?

11. The Pennsylvania school record for dental health is unique. What are the significant differences between this type of dental record and the one shown on page 110, figure 23?

12. Ten functions of the dental hygienist in public health are given in the text. What other duties can be added to these to make the dental hygienist more effective?

PART III

METHODS IN DENTAL HEALTH EDUCATION IN SCHOOLS

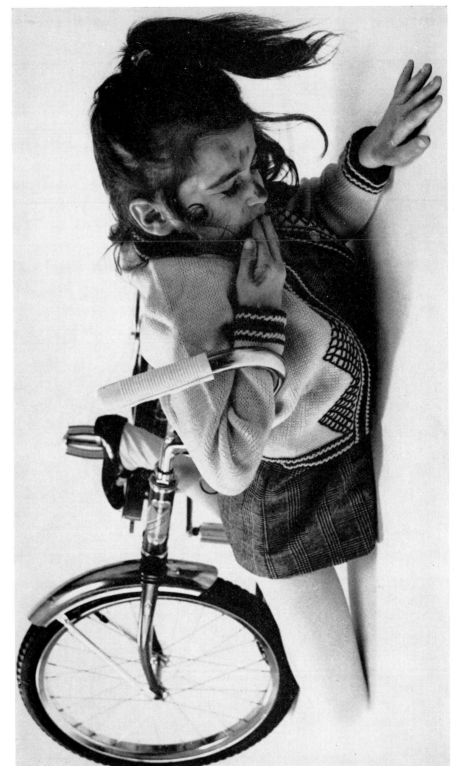

FIG. 16.—Most bicycle accidents involve injury to the teeth and jaws. Dental health should be correlated with safety instruction.

Chapter 10

Educational Concepts Applied to Dental Health Education

The Changing Purposes of Health Education in Schools

A person who takes preventive health action, as opposed to being driven by symptoms, is the person who is brought to a state of "readiness to act" by holding the three following ideas,

1. that he is susceptible to some disease, (that is, the disease is not only for others to get but he himself can be affected by it),

2. the disease is potentially serious in its effects upon him, and

3. that the course of action to overcome the disease is both available to him and effective. Preventive health behavior is a function of the resolution of conflicts among needs, motives, and perceived courses of action.

This quote is from a theory proposed by Hochbaum, Kegeles and others.* It states succinctly the philosophy upon which dental health education is predicated, emphasizing the preventive attitude which is the basis for dental health education. It can be argued that the statement is negative in its approach and that a positive approach in education is more in keeping with present-day thinking. However, as a motivating force the theory has merit. The concept of prevention is a theme which is currently being explored extensively in dentistry and it is for this reason that it seems

* Kegeles, S. Stephen,: "An Interpretation of Some Behavioral Principles in Relation to Acceptance of Dental Care," U. S. Dept. of Health, Education and Welfare, Public Health Service Publication No. 698.

pertinent to consider behavioral response to positive dental health instruction in the light of the underlying motivation which leads children to accept and practice good dental health habits.

The scope of public education has increased in many areas during the past several decades. Concern for the health of the individual during school years and as a member of the community has shown conspicuous advancement. The primary concern of education is to provide knowledge that will permit the individual to take his rightful place in society. The extent to which education has expanded to provide an adequate preparation for successful living in a democracy is indicated by the state education laws which provide for health examinations of school children.

Past Practices and Present Trends in School Health

Legislation with regard to medical inspection of school children began in Connecticut in 1899. More laws were enacted during the period from 1917 to 1924. Results of the World War I draft examinations indicated that the health of the American youth was far below the armed forces health requirements. Although school health programs expanded during this period there was little cooperative action

91

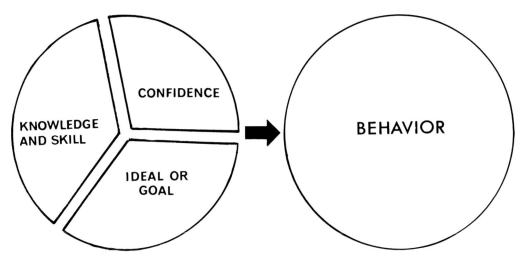

Fɪɢ. 17.—The result of knowledge and skill based on confidence and an accepted goal is a change in behavior.

among teachers and parents, the school and the community. Health classes met at any available free period on the daily schedule. Teachers were unprepared or uninterested in health instruction. Physical educators were assigned by the administrators to teach health classes but neglected them in favor of physical education activities.

When the draft rejects of World War II and the Korean War showed that there was little improvement in the physical and mental health of draftees regardless of exposure to school health education, public interest was aroused. Many of the rejected men were found to have poor vision, partial hearing, bad teeth, malnutrition and other problems directly connected with the school health service program rather than with the health instruction phase. In short, facts had been taught but health habits had not improved and the men lacked the motivation to improve their condition. As far as dental health was concerned the draft requirement was reduced to such a low level that if an individual's teeth could be repaired or dentures provided for them during enlistment so that he could eat comfortably, he was accepted. The health status of these men was a strong argument for requiring periodic health appraisal

through health examinations and dental inspections, with a complete plan for follow-up for the correction of remedial defects. Youth is entitled to grow up with a sound mind in a sound body.

Statutes permitting or requiring the examination of school children for physical defects were enacted in 1941. Now all states have either mandatory or permissive laws.

Mandatory law requires school boards to provide medical examinations. Unless the school provides the facilities and the personnel for medical examinations it may be held negligent by the courts. Mandatory law usually provides a minimum standard for examinations and often states the frequency with which the examinations must be given to the child.

Permissive law allows school boards to provide medical examinations. It lacks the power of enforcement and the school board can ignore this area of education unless some type of supervision that states specific requirements is provided in the rules and regulations that govern the school. Sometimes it is necessary for the state to withhold financial aid to schools that do not provide health safeguards for children.

Many states have specific regulations set down by the state department of education as to the length of course, course content, grade levels for teaching courses and recommended textbooks. Most states have courses of study in the form of a syllabus provided to teachers and administrators. Modification of the education laws is constantly under legislative consideration.

The relation of health to progress in education is recognized by educators. School health has become a vital part of the curriculum. The present trend in physical examinations is to give more time to each child and provide less frequent examinations. Screening examinations including those for hearing, vision and dental inspection are given by trained health workers with accurate measuring devices. Classroom teachers and health specialists including physicians, dentists, nurses and dental hygienists work together to establish the health status of each child. The school health program has become an effective service in evaluating not only the health of children but also the school environment, health instruction and health guidance for children and parents.

Health teaching is functional; it is based on the needs and interest of the child. Factual information and personal experiences are used to strengthen his understanding of the importance of health. Dental health is recognized as one of the vital needs of all children. Research has shown that there are a number of ways of protecting teeth against disease. When these are applied children can be saved from the crippling effects of tooth loss.

A serious problem still remains to be solved, that of providing complete dental treatment for all children regardless of financial status. Schools are prevented from using their funds for the correction of physical defects. Volunteer services which attempt to solve the problem by establishing dental clinics and free visits to the dentist thrive for a time but tend to disappear for lack of funds or lack of continuing motivation. Official community agencies provide some treatment services but fall short of

the need because of lack of funds and professional personnel. When dental needs are not met there is usually a lack of communication among the several agencies, the school and the parents.

Administration of School Health Programs

There are three types of health programs conducted in schools:

1. The entire program administered by the department of education.
2. The entire program administered by the department of health.
3. The *service program* administered by the department of health including supervision of communicable disease control, care of emergencies, medical and dental examinations, follow-up on health examinations, correction of defects for indigents, school nursing. The *instruction program* only is conducted by the department of education.

School and health officials are recognizing to an increasing extent the need for cooperative efforts. A number of states have representation from both the state department of health and the state department of education. In some instances a director of school health receives appointment through the joint consent of both departments. There are advantages as well as disadvantages in every type of administration of the school health program.

Arguments in favor of administration by the department of education are:

All health services can be readily made educational in character. School administrators understand educational aspects of health services better than non-school officials. There is better coordination with all educational phases of the school program. All school health activities are under one responsible head. More intensively trained and educationally oriented personnel may be employed. Health personnel can concentrate on the problems of school children.

Arguments in favor of health services administered by department of health are:

The department of health is legally responsible for control of diseases. School services can be better coordinated into the

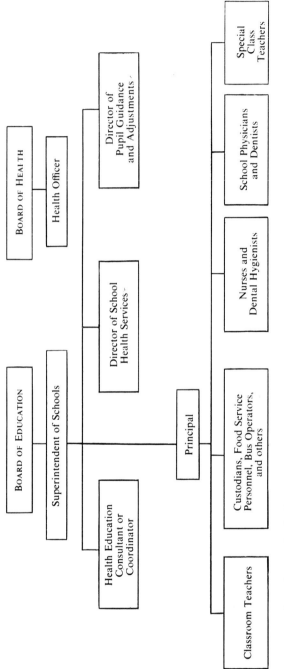

Fig. 18.—When these individuals function in a school the principal is the immediate administrative authority. In the performance of their functions there is a consultative and cooperative responsibility with the health officer and with all groups indicated as being directly responsible to the principal.

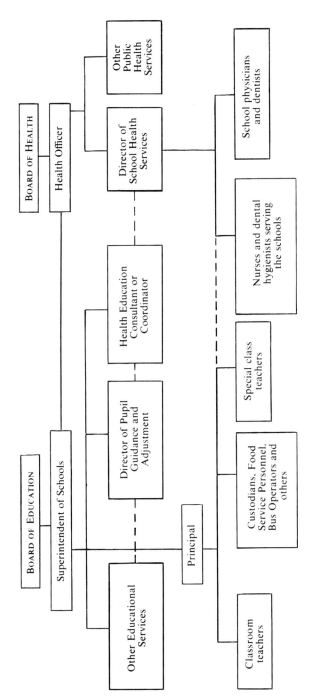

Fig. 19.—When any individual functions in a single school the principal is the immediate administrative authority. In the performance of the functions of the personnel indicated there is consultative and cooperative responsibility between the personnel operating under the superintendent of schools and the health officer. The latter's functions may include control of sanitation, prevention and control of communicable diseases, health examinations, contacts with home, intensive and planned follow-up of defects, first aid and emergency care and health supervision of physical education and athletics. (Figs. 18 and 19 reproduced from "Health Education" 4th Edition, National Education Association.)

public health programs. Community nurses and other professional personnel may have better home contacts than those working exclusively in schools. Medical services should be under medical supervision. All private schools must be serviced by the department of health and duplicate organizations are wasteful.

Figures 18 and 19 show administration of the school health program under the department of education and under the department of health.

Educational Principles and Procedures as Applied to Dental Health Education

The school's objective is the education of the whole child. Basic principles which have been formulated for health education apply to dental health.

1. *Effective health education is an integral part of the curriculum.* Dental health education should receive prime consideration within the health program since it concerns every child and has changing implications as he develops.

2. *Health is a way of living and is a part of every child's experiences in school, in the home and in the community.* Dental health is a vital part of daily living. It requires habit formation as an integral part of body cleanliness. The home provides daily toothbrushing and proper nutrition while the school provides authentic facts upon which the home regimen is based.

3. *To be effective, health information, habits and attitudes must be acquired in meaningful experiences.* Dental inspections provide an educative situation in which the child learns the condition of his own teeth. He may enter into classroom discussions that motivate him to seek dental treatment. He learns that the dentist is his friend and that regular dental visits will prevent pain and loss of teeth.

4. *The objective is the most vital and best health possible for each child.* The application of preventive measures provides a stimulating force for obtaining the best dental health in terms of teaching a

good toothbrushing technique, requiring regular dental examinations and treatment, topical application of fluorides and the restriction of free sugars in the diet.

5. *Health education programs are planned in relation to the growth patterns and the health needs of children at various age levels.* A graded curriculum in dental health instruction that recognizes the areas of interest, the conditions of growth and the dental needs is correlated with the health and safety programs. Dental safety is taught along with safety in the school environment, especially in the gymnasium and in the shop. Many accidents to teeth can be avoided if hazardous situations are recognized and discussed.

6. *Health instruction is closely related to and utilizes the provisions for healthful school living and the health services.* Nutrition and dental health are closely allied. The school lunch and the cafeteria can be a proving ground and experimental laboratory for the correction of poor food habits, particularly in restricting free sugars. The dental inspection conducted on a regular basis and closely followed by a re-check for corrections is a strong motivating force for learning by direct personal experience.

7. *Many experiences in the school, especially in social studies and science, provide opportunities for the development of desirable attitudes related to health.* Social studies may include the topic of fluoridation of the communal water supply. The value of prevention and how to reduce dental decay is learned. Children meet the challenge of adverse opinion and they come to rational conclusions concerning the use of public funds for this purpose. Children are the pioneers who influence parents to accept and promote fluoridation. Science classes teach the process of dental decay and the action of fluorides on teeth.

8. *Improved behavior toward good emotional and physical health practices is the ultimate goal; understanding and attitudes are necessary as the bases of behavior.* An understanding of dental health comes with

the knowledge of tooth structure and function; the ravages to which teeth are exposed and the means of combating these conditions. If the teacher accepts the periodic dental health inspection as an important privilege provided by the school as part of the progress toward better health, then the children will accept her attitude and place an equal amount of importance on the experience.

9. *A good program utilizes as many behavioral situations as possible.* The teacher and the children should think of dental health as a matter of conduct, not as content of instruction (facts to be learned): "I'd rather see a sermon than hear one any day, for I may misunderstand you and the high advice you give; but there is no misunderstanding how you act and how you live." The teacher who comes to school with a clean mouth and a healthy set of teeth is setting the pattern of behavior that she expects from her pupils. Regular visits to the dentist are a dental health activity she shares with her children.

10. *The environment for health education is broader than the curriculum.* It extends to the buildings, equipment, administration, and the entire school life.

11. *Special health periods devoted to direct health teaching should be determined by special needs or as the outcome of some school activity.* Much has been said about the role of the classroom teacher as the individual responsible for the health teaching in the elementary grades. In this age of specialization, a teacher can no longer be expected to know all the answers concerning health that arise in her classroom. She needs direction and guidance from health specialists who have sufficient background to answer with authority and with scientific facts. The dental hygienist is a special health educator who can provide guidance in dental health. She has a thorough background of scientific education, but she should be able to convey her knowledge in lay terms. Direct teaching of dental health facts will provide the teacher with a framework of information upon which she can plan further class activities.

12. *Evaluation of the health program and pupil progress should be in terms of improved physical, mental, moral and social behavior and the opportunities provided for healthful practices.* Dental health is an area that can be measured in terms of pupil progress. Daily health habits are evaluated by the cleanliness of each child's mouth and teeth. Healthful diet habits can be measured by the reduction in the incidence of dental caries coincident with the reduction of sugars in the diet. If the child's primary teeth are saved until the proper age and if children graduate with a full set of permanent teeth, it is evident that each child is accepting dental treatment and practicing good dental hygiene.

13. *The entire school personnel has the responsibility for taking advantage of the many opportunities for increasing good health habits and attitudes.* Incidental dental health teaching in the daily classroom routine challenges the creativity of the teacher. Enthusiasm for better dental health depends largely on the value placed on it by the teacher. It can be an important part of daily living or it can be ignored to the destruction of the teeth of the school child. Excellent opportunities exist for incidental teaching in science, social studies and in home economics classes. Creative teaching never reaches the point of saturation.

Examples to illustrate each principle have been stated. Further discussion of the topics of dental health will be developed later in the text.

Competencies and Concepts in Dental Health

The first chapter of the text provided a general understanding of what is meant by health education. The theory of teaching through "key concepts" was explained. It is appropriate at this point to analyze exactly what is meant by competencies and concepts as they relate to dental health. The State Office of Education of the State

Table 5.   Competencies and Concepts in Dental Health Education
Kindergarten through Sixth Grade*

Competency 1.   *Appreciate Growth and Function of Dental Structures*

Concepts: Primary Grades

1. Teeth have many uses
2. Kinds and numbers of teeth vary with age
3. Teeth have structure

Concepts: Intermediate Grades

1. Teeth contribute to general well-being
2. Kinds and number of teeth vary with age
3. Parts of teeth have specific functions

Competency 2.   *Know and Use Information Concerning Causes, Prevention and Correction of Dental Disorders*

Concepts: Primary Grades

1. Daily care promotes dental health
2. Foods affect teeth
3. Dentists help to maintain healthful teeth
4. Safety practices can prevent dental accidents

Concepts: Intermediate Grades

1. Regular personal care promotes dental health
2. Good diet contributes to dental health
3. Regular dental supervision helps control dental disorders
4. Accidents to teeth require immediate dental attention

Competency 3.   *Accept Responsibility for Meeting Community Dental Needs*

Concepts: Primary Grades

1. Community resources provide help for dental care

Concepts: Intermediate Grades

1. Know and use community resources for dental care

Competency 4.   *Discriminate as a Consumer of Dental Information, Products and Services*

Concepts: Primary Grades

1. Advertising affects the choice of dental products

Concepts: Intermediate Grades

1. Dental neglect is expensive for the individual
2. There are many factors which influence choices of products and services

---

* State of Washington, State Office of Education, Olympia, Washington.

of Washington provides an outline called "Health Education Guide to Better Health."

Health Knowledge, Attitudes, Practices and Skills

Concepts and competencies are implemented by an understanding of how to communicate knowledge or facts about dental health; how to develop health attitudes; how to motivate health practices, and finally, how to help the child acquire health skills.

The most important outcome of health education is the development and practice of desirable habits or behavior. In dental health this outcome is particularly important, as teeth deteriorate at such a rapid rate that desirable habits of daily care are most important. That is to say, proper care of the teeth originates with the individual and his pattern of habits such as brushing his teeth after eating; refraining from using the teeth in undesirable ways, and pernicious habits; taking the responsibility for regular dental care by the family dentist; and using every means of preventing the loss of teeth by disease or accident.

Toothbrushing, the daily habit of most people, must be learned by children. It is not a simple task for them and it requires the development of a number of educational outcomes in order to assure proficiency. These outcomes are defined and illustrated in the text by using toothbrushing as an example of a desirable health habit to be learned.

Health knowledge must precede all other goals in order to reach good dental health habits and behavior. Knowledge is the result of learning facts and procedures that help the individual to know *what* to do in a given situation and that give him sufficient knowledge of *why* he should react in a definite manner. Knowledge is obtaining facts and information, understanding, awareness, insight, reason and comprehension.

Knowledge is the sum of the individual's experiences, whether they be acquired from books, lectures and demonstrations or from direct contact experiences such as having the teeth cleaned or having a cavity filled. But knowledge cannot depend entirely on individual experience. A regular body of knowledge, commonly called *subject matter content*, must be obtained in an orderly fashion. Mankind would not have progressed very far if each generation had to depend solely upon knowledge acquired through direct experiences; instead, man has learned to benefit from the store of tested and proved knowledge. Scientific knowledge has been accumulating through the ages and it is from this source that children learn to accept certain truths without individual experimentation or the trial-and-error method of learning.

Knowledge in health education is, therefore, the type that stimulates and serves as a motivating force. It permits the child to make the proper responses, which he has learned in school, to situations outside of the classroom. Again in applying this concept to dental health, the child may learn how and when to brush his teeth the proper way, but he may not have the facilities to do so in school. He therefore learns to carry this knowledge into the home situation and to respond with the proper care of his teeth as a self-discipline.

Children need to know an exact method of brushing the teeth. It must be taught step by step, from wetting the brush and applying the dentifrice to cleaning the brush and replacing it in the proper receptacle. Each step must be described and demonstrated according to a definite plan. One of several methods may be used, but once initiated, only one method should be adhered to if habit formation is to follow.

Knowledge does not guarantee correct conduct unless it is based on learning experiences of some type, either vicarious or direct. If this concept is true, then those who argue that health teaching must be incidental to all learning fail to understand that unless a body of knowledge is planned and received in a form compatible with the individual's ability to comprehend, less than the desired motivation will result. There will be no transfer of learning from other subject areas.

Health attitudes are the reactions of the individual to the learning he has acquired. It is the state of mental and emotional readiness to accept what is known to be good and to reject that which is injurious. Attitudes are defined as preferences, likes and dislikes, values, feelings, and on a higher level, conscience or philosophy. Attitudes form the basis for behavior. If the individual's attitudes toward dental health are known, it is possible to predict the life of his teeth, within reasonable limits. If the mouth and teeth are kept free of fermentable debris the greater part of each day, it is reasonable to believe that the incidence of dental decay will be reduced; gingivitis will not progress where the stimulation of thorough toothbrushing is a daily routine. If dental treatment is received at regular intervals, there will be no loss of teeth and periodontal disease will in most instances be avoided.

Individual attitudes are acquired. They develop as the result of living in a certain environment. Attitudes may develop slowly through the long process of education or they may come suddenly as the result of an intense experience. The first experience of the child in a dental office should be conditioned by some knowledge of what he is to expect. Suppose that his first experience is to be the cleaning of his teeth. He should know that even though he brushes his teeth daily it is important that his teeth be cleaned by a dentist or dental hygienist at certain intervals to remove deposits and stains which the toothbrush cannot reach. His first visit should be a pleasant experience if his attitude toward dental treatment is to be a positive one. A bad experience might mean that the child will not accept dental treatment and will avoid all efforts to treat his teeth, with the result that he may lose them early in life.

Unfortunately, many attitudes are learned from sources less reliable than the school and it is these attitudes which must be broken down and replaced by others. For example, the antagonistic attitude of some members of a community toward the fluoridation of drinking water to prevent dental cavities may adversely influence parents so that their children may be deprived of its benefits. Forceful, enthusiastic dental health education in schools can bring about changes in poor attitudes which may have been learned through unreliable sources.

Attitudes, particularly in regard to health practices, are acquired early in life. Teachers and parents have the most influence in developing the desired attitudes, but the child also needs to be challenged in order to create for himself a set of values. If he accepts only the values of his peer groups he cannot make intelligent decisions when he is left to his own devices. Questions about dental health should be treated seriously for the child is seeking to establish his own attitudes by clarification of his factual learning. Every question deserves a clearly worded, concise answer.

Health practices are the actions that result from health knowledge and health attitudes. Dental health practices are the result of continuous use of health facts until they become fixed as habits. A habit is said to be a fixed or established response to daily situations which involve little mental activity. Habits continue not through inertia or lack of thought but rather through the daily strengthening of good attitudes. This explains the reason for a continuous program of dental health in schools. Unless there are constant reminders, emphasis and renewed motivation, there will be a gradual back-sliding in good

dental health habits in the home and a decrease in number of the regular dental appointments. Dental treatment is not pleasant at best and it takes constant reminders to persuade children that good dental health can be obtained only by constant vigilance and continuing daily the dental health practices learned in school.

Unfortunately, good dental health practices do not always show immediate results and a child who brushes his teeth may nevertheless fall prey to dental disease. The challenge for educators is to keep good dental health foremost in health goals by persistent instruction and demands that require good dental health practices.

Health skills as they relate to health education are activities that are learned through instruction. Skill in performing certain health acts such as brushing the teeth according to a certain technique is the application of knowledge. One may be able to describe a desirable method of toothbrushing, but unless the teeth are brushed by this method so that they are free of debris, the skill has not been learned. Skills are on-going or progressive. Children like to do better each time the skills they have just learned, so it is pertinent to permit practice immediately after instruction. Toothbrush drills in schools teach a skill, but they are of little benefit unless the parents supervise the activity at home and see to it that children brush all tooth surfaces in a very definite pattern so that a desirable habit is formed. Time spent with the child during the skill-practice period at home will mean a cleaner mouth for the child and improved ability in toothbrushing as time passes. Parents must supplement the school in teaching skills.

Motivation is greatest immediately after the instruction is given, but it must be renewed at frequent intervals during the learning years if skills are to improve. Dental health cannot be taught in any one grade and abandoned thereafter for it will then fall into disuse and disregard. It is for this reason that special dental health edu-

Unit 1. Personal Health	Unit 2. Growth and Development	Unit 3. Safety Education	Unit 4. Disease Prevention
Proper toothbrushing	Tooth structure	Types of tooth accidents	Prevention and protection
Adequate dental treatment	Tooth forms	Areas of prevention	Topical fluorides
Your teeth for life	Supporting tissues	Undesirable mouth habits	Disclosing wafers
Individual responsibility	Primary and permanent teeth	Prevention of accidents in gymnasium, shop and games	Orthodontics
Consumer education	Mechanism of chewing and swallowing	Mouthguards, use and abuse	Effects of tooth loss
Analysis of advertising	Occlusion		Periodontal disease
Dentifrices, mouthwashes, tooth whiteners			

Unit 5. Community Health	Unit 6. Mental and Social Health	Unit 7. Nutrition	Unit 8. Stimulants and Depressants
Resources for dental treatment	Psychological effects of bad teeth	Adequate diet	Symptoms of drug addiction seen in the mouth
Voluntary and official agencies	Good teeth and self-confidence	Role of nutrients in dental health	Results of malnutrition on teeth
Water fluoridation	Social standards of dental health	Diet analysis	Role of the dentist and dental hygienist in discovering drug addiction
Financing dental services	Job success related to good teeth	Reasons for restriction of free sugars	
Community responsibilities	Accepting dental treatment without fear	What constitutes a good breakfast, lunch, snacks and dinner	
Care of indigents	Mouth and teeth are sensory organs	Detergent foods	
Head Start programs			
Group insurance for dental health			

Fig. 20. Health education curriculum units showing dental health instruction correlation.

cators have been employed in a number of states. They are licensed dental hygienists with special education in teaching techniques. It is their main duty to see that every child has a knowledge of dental facts suited to his period of mental development; that he and his parents have the benefit of guidance in reference to dental health problems and that re-check for correctable defects is made soon after the school inspection. These are motivating forces which keep dental health practices alive and which supplement and enforce knowledge of dental health facts. There should be a steady flow of information throughout the school life of the child to keep his interest (motivation) and his attitudes reaching for better dental health.

Correlation of Dental Health Instruction in the Curriculum of Health Education

It has been shown that a unit in dental health should be included in a health curriculum in order to insure an authentic body of knowledge. However, it is also quite necessary that dental health be interrelated to other units of study within the health curriculum. In outline, this concept is shown in figure 20.

Questions for Review and Discussion

1. The Hochbaum-Kegeles theory is a philosophy of fear. Explain why it is acceptable as a motivating force in promoting dental health.

2. Numerous changes have taken place in school health programs. In what areas has the greatest change occurred?

3. Explain why dental health habits and skills add to a child's sense of security.

4. List the 13 principles on which a health program is based and add a dental health item other than those mentioned

under each principle (open book question).

5. Give your own definition of the following as they relate to dental health education: concept, competency, motivation, skill, and habit.

6. All state education laws contain either permissive or mandatory laws concerning health examinations of school children. Which of these is most effective Why?

7. What evidence is there that classroom teachers are not prepared to present dental health facts without the assistance of professional dental personnel?

8. Did you have dental health instruction in elementary school? In high school? Was it effective in helping you to establish better dental health habits? Discuss and compare your experiences with other members of your class.

9. Discuss fully one concept under each competency as suggested in the Washington State listing.

10. Unit 6, "Mental and Social Health," is a very important topic in health education at the present time. Choose one item under this heading and explore it at length.

Selected Readings

Anderson, C. L.: SCHOOL HEALTH PRACTICE, C. V. Mosby Co., St. Louis, 2nd Edition, 1960, p. 243.

Cornacchia, H. J., Staton, W. M., Irwin, L. W.: HEALTH IN ELEMENTARY SCHOOLS, C. V. Mosby Co., St. Louis, 3rd Edition, 1970, p. 206.

Fodor, J. T., Dalis, G. T.: HEALTH INSTRUCTION: THEORY AND APPLICATION, Lea & Febiger, Philadelphia, 1966, p. 54.

Nemir, A.: SCHOOL HEALTH PROGRAM, W. B. Saunders Co., Philadelphia, 1970. p. 356.

Stoll, F. A., Catherman, J. L.: DENTAL HEALTH EDUCATION, Lea & Febiger, Philadelphia, 3rd Edition, 1967, p. 214.

Student Teaching Handbook, Dental Hygiene (Mimeograph), University of Bridgeport, School of Dental Hygiene, Bridgeport, Conn.

Chapter 11

Planning the Dental Health Program in Schools

Defining the Problem

Effective application of the measures for the control of disease depends to a great extent upon knowledge of the *manner* in which disease occurs in population groups. Collection of information concerning the disease is, therefore, a pre-requisite to effective planning for a control program*

The survey method of collecting data produces the amount and type of data suited for analyzing the dental health needs of school children. Selected items are obtained which help to determine the kind of dental health program most appropriate for a given school situation. Individual case histories are recorded and at a later date these data can be used for research studies. This method of compiling information is called "case-finding technique."

Planning a dental health program also requires a statement of objectives. The goals to be achieved are determined in relation to the available resources. The formulation of new objectives is an on-going process as the program is constantly modified. The objectives of the dental health program are directly related to the broad objectives of the school. Planning is a cooperative undertaking. All the resources of the faculty, administration and facilities are utilized.

Objectives and Purposes

The American Dental Association has adopted the following objectives as a guide.

"The control of dental caries and other disease of the mouth and teeth is best accomplished during childhood.

1. Help every American appreciate the importance of a healthy mouth.

2. Help every American appreciate the relationship of dental health and appearance.

3. Encourage good dental health practices including personal mouth hygiene, professional care, proper diet and good oral habits.

4. Enlist the aid of all groups and agencies interested in the promotion of health.

5. Correlate dental health with generalized health programs.

6. Stimulate the development of resources for making dental care available to all children and youth.

7. Stimulate all dentists to perform dental health services for children.†

Survey of the School District

When a dental health program is to be initiated in a school system it should be established upon the results of a survey of the school district. The survey should

---

* Pelton, W. F., Wisan, J. M.: DENTISTRY IN PUBLIC HEALTH, W. B. Saunders Co., Philadelphia, 2nd Edition, 1955, p. 11.

† Dental Health Program for Elementary and Secondary Schools, Council on Dental Health, American Dental Association.

be made by those who are to be responsible for the program, the dental hygienist, the supervising dentist, the health coordinator and the school health council. Ideally a dentist and a dental hygienist who both have a dental background supplemented by courses in education and public health are the best qualified to supervise the survey. Some of the areas of investigation are:

1. A survey of the general population to determine **A.**, the distribution and location of native and foreign minority groups in order to understand their customs and beliefs. Information can be obtained through several sources including the office of the administrator of the school; local government agencies where census figures are kept; local churches; racial groups and their organizations. **B.**, the financial status of various groups within the community. Information in this area will help to formulate policies relating to dental treatment planning. Sources of information are industries and employment agencies; real estate values in various neighborhoods; the number of home owners compared to renters. The type of population, whether itinerant or permanent, has a direct bearing on the type of dental health program necessary. **C.**, the school population census and the estimated fluctuation of school population within the next ten years. A school census is taken each summer in most school districts. All factors that affect the school populations such as birth rates, transfers into and out of the district; increase and decrease in general population; new buildings, homes, factories and stores are studied. School boards watch these trends closely as guides to future development of the schools. Records are kept in the superintendent's office. **D.**, social agency facilities, official and voluntary, should be known as possible sources of financial aid to the dental health program. A spot map showing the office location of each dentist and clinic is a means of quick reference and will save much time after the program is in operation. It should be revised from time to time

as new facilities and new dentists settle in the community.

2. Past programs that include dental health in the schools should be reviewed and evaluated. The parts of these programs which have been effective should be retained; ineffective efforts should be discarded. Thus, mistakes are not repeated. The administrator can provide historical records of past procedures and programs.

3. Records and reports of the general health program as well as the dental phase should be thoroughly read and accomplishments and failures noted. An individual record of each child is usually kept. These are in the form of cumulative records as the child progresses. They provide full information about the child's health as well as his academic achievement record. The dental health record should be a part of the complete health record. A separate dental health record in more detail is usually kept in the dental health room for immediate reference.

4. Conferences. A thorough understanding of the objectives and purposes of the dental health program should be discussed at conferences of all health and instructional personnel so that there is an agreement on procedures and general cooperation. Many misunderstandings can be avoided if these conferences are held during the planning stage. Parents and pupils are brought into the planning after the fundamentals have been agreed upon by the teaching and professional staffs.

5. Financial support. It is important that separate funds be allotted to the dental health program. A special item in the school budget earmarked for dental health will avoid confusion with other health items. Dental health programs will be organized largely on the amount of funds available. Ambitious programs without adequate financing are doomed to failure. The amount of the budget makes a vast difference in the goals to be accomplished. A study of the factors that constitute the dental health budget shows that the largest

sums are spent for salaries of personnel such as dentists, dental hygienists and clerical help. The next largest sum is used for equipment and supplies. Less frequently, some schools show an allotment for dental treatment of indigent children. Gathering of data on the dental health status of the child is discussed fully in the section, "Appraisal of Individual Dental Health."

Parts of the Dental Health Education Program

There are three phases in the dental health education program: (a) dental health instruction, (b) dental health services and (c) dental treatment including preventive procedures.

An accepted definition for health education applies equally to dental health: "The sum of all the experiences which favorably influence practices, attitudes, and knowledge relating to health." Each phase of the program can be carried to completion only when there is an interdependence with the other two phases. There are no clear-cut lines of demarcation among the three. Instruction will be found in the service phase and in the treatment phase. Some of the most beneficial instruction takes place in the dental chair during treatment. The dental inspection is not simply a case-finding technique, but also an opportunity for health guidance and counseling. The re-check and follow-up procedures can be part of the instructional phase, particularly if the classroom teacher assumes responsibility for some of the follow-up for dental corrections.

Health Guidance Defined

Health counseling consists of the procedures for helping pupils and parents to understand the nature and significance of conditions revealed by dental inspections and to solve dental health problems. It is of little value to discover, year after year, that a child has dental defects if nothing is done to correct them. Little progress is made if the advantages of prevention are

discussed but neither the school nor the community makes it possible for the child to obtain preventive care.

Health guidance applies to dental health as a process of developing attitudes and ideals concerning dental health. The child is made aware of his physical nature and the need to follow certain rules of health which will correct his dental deficiencies and provide for future good dental health. It is an effort to instill good habits and attitudes based on self-recognition of needs and the importance of meeting them. Health guidance is the opposite of accepting blindly that which is taught as truth without commitment to changing attitudes.

The Dental Health Service Program

The service program in dental health is based largely on individual guidance. Determining the dental health status of each child in relation to his school group, his family unit and his community at large is a function of the service phase.

The component parts of the service program for dental health in schools are:

Periodic Dental Inspection:
Annual inspection for all children; special period of inspection for absentees; consultation for students re-admitted after absence due to toothache; consultation for students who complain of dental pain or discomfort; consultation for students who need release time for dental appointments; conference with parents to obtain the dental history, and medical history when essential; information supplied by grade teacher through daily health observations; information about general health supplied by the school nurse.

Records:
Identifying date: Name, address, parents' names; parents' occupations; family physician and family dentist. School attended, classroom number and grade, age at yearly inspection, significant items of family history.
Dental health status: date of inspection, record of dental defects, treatment received and needed in terms of decayed, missing and filled teeth (DMF), type of occlusion (good, fair or poor), mouth hygiene (stains, calculus, condition of gingiva), use of the toothbrush (after eating, daily, occasionally).
Recording of dental status on cumulative health record.

Reports:
Monthly and annual reports to administrators with copy to the supervising dentist.
Notification to parent of need for dental care; list of pupils in need of dental treatment to teacher, nurse or other health specialist.
Referral of indigent children for dental treatment to official and voluntary agencies.

Follow-up Program:
Re-check for correction of remediable defects through additional dental inspection; review of dental health record; conferences with teachers, health personnel and family dentist; home visits or visits to school by parents; group conferences with parents, teachers and administrators; re-check for corrections.

Emergency Care:
First aid in dental emergencies; excuses from school for emergency care by dentist in case of accidents to teeth or toothache; contacts with teachers, nurses, parents and dentist in case of dental emergencies.

Dental Prophylaxis:
As an educative experience; preparing children to accept dental treatment; as a service to indigent children prior to dental treatment; as an adjunct to regular dental care.

Evaluation:
Observation of individual and group dental health habits; survey for corrections obtained; completion of health records; interpretation of findings to administrators, teachers and other health personnel; study of program strength and weakness; continuous process of improvement through periodic evaluation of procedures and objectives; evaluation of pupil progress in dental health practices.

Periodic Dental Inspections

The detection of dental disease is a function of the dental hygienist or the dentist, rather than of the physician, nurse or classroom teacher. Byrd says,

> The early detection of dental disorders through school screening programs is just as logical as similar programs for the detection of children with losses of vision or hearing or any other kind of health handicap that may impair the learning capacity of the child.[*]

School health examinations are conducted in fragments by many different persons. An adequate appraisal of the child's health is facilitated when there is a pooling of classroom observations by the teacher, by re-

---

[*] Byrd, O. E.: SCHOOL HEALTH ADMINISTRATION, W. B. Saunders Co., Philadelphia, 1964, p. 208.

ports from the family physician and dentist, by school nurse inspections, by results of psychological tests and by information from many other sources.

In the school health examinations there are ten primary parts:

1. The health history
2. Physical examination
3. Emotional appraisal
4. Vision screening
5. Screening for hearing disorders
6. Speech appraisal
7. Dental health inspection
8. Growth records
9. Posture appraisal
10. Special procedures (chest X ray, tuberculin test, etc.)

The dental inspection is an aspect of health appraisal and should be conducted mainly for educational and appraisal purposes. During the dental inspection, the child should learn the general condition of his own dental health and the reasons for the procedures which are to follow the inspection. The dental inspection should be conducted in a friendly but professional atmosphere. The child should learn to respect the procedure and the persons who carry it out as important to his own health. He should also be aware that he is receiving respect as an individual.

There is added value in the dental inspection when parents are informed, either during the inspection by being present or directly after the inspection by notification in writing. Information and guidance for parents at this time should include an evaluation of the child's dental health practices at home and an explanation of the need for correcting dental defects.

All health examinations are more fruitful for the individual child if they are preceded by a classroom activity which gives information about the method of conducting the experience and the learning that should result. In this way, the child becomes an active participant in the dental inspection rather than a passive subject, and so, he will not feel that his privacy is being exploited. If proper orientation to inspection procedures is planned, possible criticism by parents may be avoided. Most criticism comes from lack of information about what is being done for the good and welfare of children in school.

Dental inspections as differentiated from dental examinations may be provided at regular intervals. The results of such inspections may be used (1) to estimate group dental needs, (2) to facilitate community planning to meet the needs and (3) to provide a base line for evaluating the dental health program. School dental inspections should be made by a dentist or dental hygienist using a mouth mirror and explorer.

Benefits of Dental Inspections

The American Dental Association states that the dental inspection conducted in the schools has the following benefits.

1. It serves as a basis for school dental health instruction.

2. It builds a positive attitude in the child toward the dentist and dental care.

3. The child is motivated to seek adequate professional care.

4. Teachers, students, dentists and others concerned with school dental health may use the dental inspection as a fact finding experience.

5. Base line and cumulative data for evaluation of the school dental health program are made available.

6. It provides information as to the status of dental needs, leading to the support of a sound dental health program.

Limitations of School Dental Inspections

1. Unless the purpose of the dental inspection in school is understood, parents tend to depend on it rather than to seek periodic examination, including X rays, in the dentist's office.

2. The primary purpose of motivating parents and children to seek and obtain regular dental care by the family dentist is

not fulfilled unless a definite follow-up is provided.

3. It is desirable for parents to be present during dental examinations. This procedure is not always feasible in school inspections.

4. Children should acquire, early in life, the habit of visiting the family dentist regularly for examination and care. Some school inspections may tend to discourage rather than to promote the development of this habit of personal initiative.

There has been much criticism about medical and dental examinations in schools during the past decade. The consensus is that medical and dental examinations in schools are not diagnostic in nature, but rather case-finding techniques. The continued use of these practices is advised for the purpose of stimulating parents to seek the professional services of the family dentist and the family physician. The inspections in school serve to motivate the child to better health attitudes and habits. The evaluation of a dental health program in terms of corrections and guidance depends largely on the data obtained during health appraisal inspections. Dental inspections help to determine the content of health instruction and serve as a medium of evaluation in health teaching.

The term "inspection" is preferred as indicating a cursory observation of the mouth and teeth of each child, as contrasted to the thorough examination as conducted in a dental office. The term "screening" is often used in place of "inspection." The dental inspection includes a clinical observation of mouth hygiene, the condition of the teeth and surrounding mucosa. The purpose of the inspection is not to count the number of cavities, as dental X rays would be required to locate all such lesions, nor to suggest methods of treatment. These decisions rest with the family dentist.

The method of inspection will vary with the facilities available, but there is a minimum standard below which no dental inspection should fall. The following minimum standards are recommended.

Types of Dental Inspections

Type 1. Complete examination including case history and diet information consists of using the mouth mirror and explorer, adequate illumination, thorough X-ray survey and, when necessary, percussion, pulp vitality tests, transillumination, study models and laboratory tests. This type of examination can only be obtained in well-equipped dental offices and dental clinics. A complete examination is given when a new patient is admitted to the office or clinic.

Type 2. Limited examination, using mouth mirror and explorer, adequate illumination, posterior bite-wing X rays and, when indicated, apical X rays. The limited examination is usually indicated at each period of recall for dental treatment and prophylaxis.

Type 3. Inspection, using mouth mirror and explorer and adequate illumination. School inspections also include the recording of adequate data to provide identification of dental needs for each child.

Type 4. Screening, using tongue depressor and available illumination. Screening is employed by physicians and nurses during general physical examinations. Screening is so superficial that it may be misleading rather than informative. Screening for dental defects should never be employed by teachers or other untrained personnel.

The Legality of School Health Services

The court has established clearly the legal right of the school to provide school health services for the pupil. As dental inspections are included in these services, the courts would uphold the right of a school system to perform such inspections. This is shown by a number of legal decisions on a variety of problems related to school health services.

It must not be assumed, however, that the courts have given the schools unrestricted authority in this field. Definite limitations have been indicated. Since the school exists as an educational institution, it is to be expected that school health services related to the educability of the individual might receive legal approbation. This proves to be the case. There is sharp curtailment, however, in school activities that might be considered purely medical or surgical, such as the establishing of a school dental clinic.

There appears to be less litigation concerning health instruction in the schools than is related to other aspects of the school health program, perhaps because there is less threat to life and limb from instruction than from negligence on the part of the school or its employees in respect to accident or disease. It may be that since every state has some compulsory feature regarding the teaching of healthful living there is less tendency to challenge the right of the school to provide learning experience in the curriculum related to this field.

Recommended Standards for the Health Suite

Approved standards for the health suite, including space measurements, furnishings and equipment recommended by the State Education Board of New York State (Fig. 21), serve as a base line for adequate accommodations and space for dental inspections. The dental health room is part of the total health suite. The choice of location is important. As the suite is used for individual counseling, interviews with parents and small conferences, it should be located near the main entrance of the building, close to the administrative office. The health suite should be away from unnecessary noises such as those emanating from boiler rooms, shops and gymnasiums. It should suggest health rather than sickness; therefore, an atmosphere of cheerfulness and informality should prevail. The health suite is not a clinic, so the hospital atmosphere should be avoided. Colors add to the general atmosphere. Floors should be of materials which are easy to clean.

In addition to the suggested floor plan, running water should be available adjacent to the dental chair. A good light for illuminating the mouth should be provided at the dental inspection chair. A supply of mouth mirrors and explorers sufficient to complete the inspection of at least two entire classes

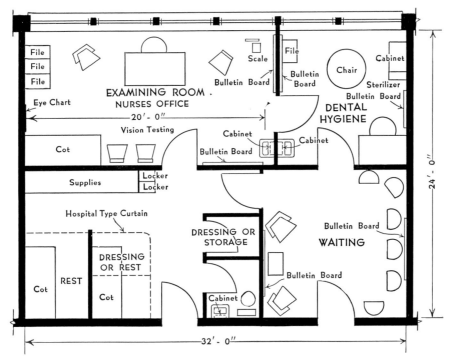

FIG 21.—Suggested health suite for over 800 pupils. Scale ⅛″ = 1′-0″.

will speed up the work. Charts for dental health data should be suited to the needs of the particular program, and sufficient quantities should be ordered in advance to allow for a complete record of each child.

Evaluating the Service Program

The school dental health program is intended to be a program lasting over a period of years rather than a one-time fact-finding effort. There is little need to obtain information that has already been found and recorded for significant sampling in a similar situation. For instance, the DMFS (adult caries index) and def (caries rate for primary teeth) rates for any school system will probably be very nearly the same as the national rates. However, to know whether teeth are missing by extraction is important. This item of evaluation will indicate whether dental care is obtained early enough to save teeth. It is important to know whether cavities are being filled, but it is neither necessary nor advisable to

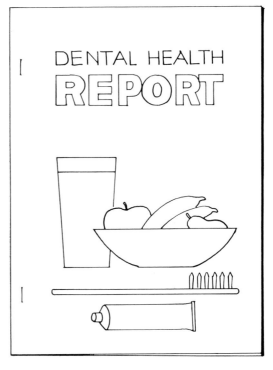

FIG. 22.

COLUMBIA UNIVERSITY SCHOOL OF DENTAL AND ORAL SURGERY,
COURSES FOR DENTAL HYGIENISTS

Name

Address

Parent or
Guardian

Occupation

ECONOMIC STATUS

A = Home Relief

B = Other Welfare Agencies

C = Cannot Afford Private Treatment

* CODE

M = Medical Center

C = Health Dept. Clinic

P = Private dentist or other clinic

School
Grade or Home Room
Date of Inspection

Teeth	Clean
	Dirty
Gums	Pink
	Red
Occlusion	Good
	Poor

Orthodontia *

Cavities	Temp
	Perm
Roots & Abceses	Temp
	Perm

Missing Perm Teeth
Under Treatment *
Work Completed *
Prophylaxis
Absent--Toothaches
Card Mailed
Home Call
Parent Conference

Fig. 23.—Dental health record form.

count the number of cavities or fillings. This item leads to a number of misunderstandings among dentists and dental health educators about which teeth should be treated and which do not need treatment. See figure 23 for the suggested form for the dental inspection with items to be recorded.

1. Dental Defects Recorded on the Chart of the Dental Record.
   a. Visible caries in deciduous and permanent teeth to determine urgency of dental treatment.
   b. Number of filled permanent and deciduous teeth to determine past dental care and incidence of decay.
   c. Number of lost permanent teeth (see Table 7 on page 114) to evaluate the dental health program as a whole in terms of the number of teeth being saved.
2. Type of Occlusion. For school health purposes it is unnecessary to use specific occlusal types. "Good" indicates that the child is not suffering from any functional disability due to occlusion; "Fair" indicates that the child must be watched as the teeth erupt; "Poor" indicates that the child is in immediate need of dental attention for the purpose of diagnosis and treatment for malocclusion.
3. Mouth Hygiene. Record the condition of the gingiva and oral mucosa: 1—normal; 2—light red, some degree of inflammation; 3—dark red, extreme degree of inflammation. Stains and calculus are rated as: 1—light; 2—moderate; 3—heavy.
   Use of the toothbrush may be recorded as: 1—thorough brushing after eating; 2—daily brushing; 3—infrequent or no brushing.
4. Anomalies. Space should be allowed on the chart for stating deviations from the normal. These may be specifically located on the dental chart. They include retained roots, supernumerary teeth, abscesses, fistulas, abnormal growths of bone and soft tissues.
   Note: When numerals are used in charting and recording, a key to the symbols should be shown on the record.

Dental inspections should be completed early in the school year in order to provide for sufficient dental appointments to complete dental treatment during the school year. Early inspection also provides a longer period for individual guidance.

Re-check inspections are the beginning of the follow-up for dental corrections. Unless there is a small number of pupils, only those who were found to have remediable dental defects should be called to the dental health room for a re-inspection. Some schools require a note from the dentist stating specifically whether dental care is started or completed. If this is the case the dentist's judgment must be accepted. The dental associations have requested that the dentist not sign a completion notice unless all treatment is finished.

A notation on the child's record should indicate that the dental treatment is "Completed," "Under Treatment," or "No Treatment."

Notations should be entered upon the dental record for each child. At the time of the re-check inspection *additional lost permanent teeth should be noted.* These lost teeth will affect the final lost permanent tooth index for the year.

In order to save time, dental conditions are usually entered on the cumulative health record at the end of the school year, principally so that the achievement results may be recorded. If the dental condition of any child must be known during the year, it may be obtained from the dental record. If a child is being neglected, it will show at the end of the year, not during the first inspection.

The children who show a record of poor mouth hygiene should be re-checked within a few days after the first inspection. Mouth hygiene is a matter of proper attitudes and habit formation as well as skill in performing the task of toothbrushing. Therefore, it is necessary to stimulate and motivate each child to take proper personal care of his teeth by regular effective brushing. The classroom teacher should be given the names of children who are not practicing good mouth hygiene. Best results can be obtained through cooperation with the classroom teacher. If children do not show improvement in a short time, the dental hygienist or other health personnel must stimulate interest by individual counseling, conferences with parents and home visits. In selected cases, a dental prophylaxis given in school is an educative means of persuading children to practice good mouth hygiene.

Preparation of Reports

In conducting a dental health program in schools, it is important to have evidence of what is happening, of changes that are occurring as the program develops. Evidence in the form of records and reports should be accumulated systematically. Records and reports become important evaluation instruments. A good set of reports may be the means of continuing a dental health program, or the lack of good progress reports may prove the undoing of a worthwhile effort.

Hints on the Format for a Report Presentation

Since reports are usually filed and kept for a number of years, they should all be the same size. Unusually large or small sheets require special handling and tend to become worn or lost. Single sheets have the same disadvantage. Therefore, a report should have some type of binding to hold it together. The attractiveness of a report begins with the cover, which should be appropriate for the type of report represented. The more formal reports need little more than a good title page. Reports to parents and to the community or a voluntary agency can use a more ornate cover that is eye-catching (see Fig. 22).

Solid pages of type are not easy to read. Think in terms of ease of reading by providing a line which does not tax the eyes of your reader. Wide margins are not wasteful; they serve to make the report more readable and provide space for comments by the readers.

Place tables, charts and graphs as close as possible to the text that describes them. Use statistics that are meaningful. Remember that large numbers are difficult to understand and most of them can be broken down into meaningful smaller numbers.

Table 6.—Dental Health Report—Schools No. 1 and 2 Comparative Percentage of Dental Corrections During Several School Years

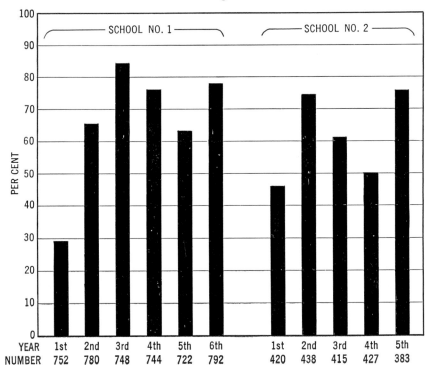

For example, the number of lost permanent teeth for 2,290 children would not have much meaning. The reader cannot tell whether this is high or low rate of loss. However, when the figure is expressed as the number of teeth lost per 100 children, it has meaning. It can be compared with statistics of other communities and with statistics of other years in the same community.

In evaluating a written report, consider:

Does the report fulfill the need for information?
Is it presented clearly so that lay people can understand it?
Has it given sufficient explanation and detail without cluttering the main points?
Will it make a good impression on those who read it?
How can it be improved in format and content at the next writing?

Table 6 indicates the trend toward better dental health through increased dental corrections. Over a period of five to six years the program has made progress toward the goal of good dental health for the school child. Because of the dental health instruction given in each grade, the adequate den-

tal treatment, methodical toothbrushing and mouth hygiene, a decrease in the rate of dental decay may be expected.

Items included in a dental health service report:

1. Comparative statistics. Several years may be reported to show the progress of the program in dental treatment (Table 6).
2. Dental health counseling.
3. Conferences, home visits and special meetings.
4. Follow-up work.
5. Resumé of instruction program.
6. Dental prophylaxis and topical fluoride treatments.
7. Recommendations such as additional personnel and equipment, supplies and financial support; ways and means of increasing home and community participation; review and revision of forms and procedures.

Some schools require a monthly report. A short form may be used as indicated in figure 24.

DENTAL HYGIENE TEACHER'S REPORT

SCHOOL_____   MONTH_____

INSPECTIONS

	Past Month	Present Month	Total

    Number of inspections
    Number with teeth in good condition
    Number with defects

FOLLOW-UP WORK
    Corrective advice cards mailed
    Parent conferences at school
    Parents contacted by telephone
    Home calls
    Letters to parents
    Pupils under treatment
    Treatment completed

EDUCATIONAL WORK—CLASSROOM
    Classroom visits
    Visual aids used

PROPHYLAXIS

_____
Dental Hygiene Teacher

Fig. 24.

Table 7.—The Number of Permanent Teeth Lost

School	Number Lost Permanent Teeth per 100 Children					Per Cent of Children with Lost Permanent Teeth				
	1st. year	2nd. year	3rd. year	4th. year	5th. year	1st. year	2nd. year	3rd. year	4th. year	5th. year
No. 1	10	5.7	15.7*	10.6	5.9	4	2	12*	7	4
No. 2.	10	10.2	9	3	8.9*	5	6	4	1	6*

* The increase in the lost permanent tooth index in school No. 1 in the third year was due to lack of dental care among the eighth grade pupils. The increase in the lost permanent tooth index in school No. 2 during the fifth year was due to the number of children enrolled in the higher grades for the first time. The method of computing the index is shown on page 114.

The Lost Permanent Tooth Index

The lost permanent tooth index is an excellent item to evaluate program progress. It is found by adding all permanent teeth indicated as extracted on all dental records.

$$\frac{\text{Number of lost teeth}}{\text{Number of children inspected}} \times 100 \text{ children} = \begin{array}{c}\text{Lost permanent}\\\text{tooth index per}\\\text{100 children.}\end{array}$$

This equation is used to obtain a whole number which has significance. The lost permanent tooth index is usually presented as a comparative statistic by showing the index for several years. It is a simple, direct indication that the program is saving teeth through effective instruction which has resulted in early and regular dental treatment.

Questions for Review and Discussion

1. Why are case-finding techniques used in preparing dental health programs in schools?

2. Why are health records, histories and cumulative records used?

3. When a dental health program is initiated in a school system, a survey of the district should be made. Select a community and secure the necessary information for an effective dental health program by using the areas of investigation suggested in the text (see page 103) (committee project). Submit a suitable report to the class.

4. State briefly the role of the other personnel (not in health) in the planning stage of the dental health program.

5. What are the principal objectives of guidance and counseling in dental health?

6. There have been strong objections at times to the dental inspection in schools, but the courts have ruled that health services in the form of screening, inspection or examination are the duty of the school. Give reasons why the dental health inspection is an important part of health appraisal.

7. Name the component parts of the service program for dental health in schools?

8. What specialized training is suggested for dental hygienists and supervising dentists who conduct dental health programs in schools?

9. What special precautions should be stressed in selecting a location for the dental health suite?

Selected Readings

Anderson, C. L.: SCHOOL HEALTH PRACTICE, Chapter 17, C. V. Mosby Co., St. Louis, 4th Edition, 1968.

Cornacchia, H. J., Staton, W. M., Irwin, L. W.: HEALTH IN ELEMENTARY SCHOOLS, Chapter 4, C. V. Mosby Co., St. Louis, 1970.

Fodor, J. T., Dalis, G. T.: HEALTH INSTRUCTION: THEORY AND APPLICATION, Chapter 4, Lea & Febiger, Philadelphia, 1968.

Nemir, A.: SCHOOL HEALTH PROGRAM, Chapter 19, W. B. Saunders Co., Philadelphia, 1970.

Weir, J. M.: "New Forms of Dental Health Education," Journal Public Health Dentistry, Fall Issue, 1970, p. 218.

Chapter 12

Improved Methods of Teaching in Dental Health

"Method is the body of educational endeavor. Educational method is as much the concern of the instructor as the mastery of subject matters used in teaching. Teaching is a combination of art and science. Science is analytical. It breaks things into parts, seeks detail and looks for causes. Art on the other hand gives meaning to science. It puts together. Science relates facts to facts; art relates facts to life."*

Teaching-learning Process

Learning takes place mostly when one *intends* to learn and *desires* to remember. Everyone recalls many of the things that happened at the "edge of attention" rather than at the "center of attention." However, unorganized learning and unguided learning cannot be depended upon to result in more than minimal and incomplete learning. A more formal type of learning must provide each child with a *frame of reference* from which he can gather factual information and apply it to a given situation in which he makes choices and decisions. This is called the process of teaching. It is formal in the sense that it is organized; it is guided and it provides accepted facts and essential principles.

Dental health instruction is effective when the conditions of learning are good

and the aim of instruction is clearly recognized. Curiosity must be aroused; information must be given and opportunities provided for practical application.

Criteria Applied to Method

A number of criteria may be applied to various methods of instruction:

1. Will the method employed promote the desired outcomes?

2. Is the method adaptable to the kind of activities involved?

3. Does the method seem feasible in relation to space, equipment, time and teaching load?

4. Is the method interesting to those being taught?

5. Do pupils have enough background information to profit by the method chosen?

6. Are new ideas tried from time to time in an effort to find the best way to organize the learning experience so that good dental health habits will result?

7. Does the method used allow opportunity for each individual to have an effective learning experience?

Guides to Dental Health Instruction Techniques

Any of the various types of teaching-learning methods may be used during the whole or only a part of a class period. Procedures should be adapted to the needs of the class and to the subject matter that is to be learned.

* Willgoose, Carl E.: HEALTH EDUCATION IN THE ELEMENTARY SCHOOL, W. B. Saunders Co., Philadelphia, 1969, p. 272.

9

Lecture Method. The lecture as a method of teaching is a formalized presentation of factual material by the teacher. The main function is to provide a foundation of understanding upon which other types of instruction may depend. For this reason, it is the most frequently used method in dental health education. Each child must know the proper rules of dental health before he can practice them. The lecture method is used to:

1. *Introduce new topics*
   Motivates and interests the child in new ideas.
   Creates a favorable mind-set toward subject matter.
   Gives direction to further activities.
   Shows how new facts relate to living.
   Relates to past experiences.
   Uses illustrations and visual aids.

2. *Summarize ideas and facts*
   Orients the thoughts of students toward desired objectives.
   Relates new facts to those already known.
   Projects thinking into action.

3. *Review*
   Brings out important facts for evaluation and discussion.
   Maintains interest by repetition of facts by using new ways of expression and new terms.
   Emphasizes important points.
   Gives students time to assimilate ideas.
   Prepares for later discussion.

Examples: Presentation of facts concerning personal dental health; the function of fluorides in water supplies; dental research and what it is doing for us.

Lecture-Demonstration Method. As the name suggests, this method combines telling with showing. The purpose of the demonstration is to set forth facts in concrete form. It is used very successfully in teaching toothbrushing. It has replaced the class laboratory sessions in schools where facilities are limited. The teacher does the demonstration; class discussion and questions follow. Students repeat the demonstration immediately or at a later session.

The chief value of the lecture-demonstration method lies in the economical use of time and in the concentration of attention. It is economical in the use of equipment; provides learning experiences that are more interesting and meaningful than an oral presentation alone. There are three steps in the lecture-demonstration method. 1., The learning problem is introduced—stimulation. 2., The demonstration develops understanding—assimilation. 3., The learned information is reinforced through the demonstration—application.

Discussion Method. Discussion is a group activity in which the students and teacher define a problem and seek its solution. The problem is analyzed, compared and evaluated. Conclusions are drawn and a plan of action formulated. This method lends itself to parent groups and high school students as an excellent means of arousing interest in dental health problems. It can also be used in modified forms in elementary grades.

There are many ways of presenting the problem, either through student or teacher leadership. Students can prepare and present facts. The teacher can introduce the topic. A resumé of facts can be a joint project of class and teacher. Special reports can be read to initiate the discussion.

The chief value of the discussion method is that it develops the student's ability to reason through problems; to accept group opinion; and to contribute personally to the discussion. While there must be leadership in order to keep the discussion pertinent to the subject under consideration, the main value to the individual is the freedom it allows in the learning process. He may accept, reject, or withhold his opinion of a group decision. Based on what he has heard during discussion, he may make whatever personal attitude changes he feels are workable in his particular situation.

The discussion method is most valuable in dental health education when professional and parent groups are concerned about the unmet needs of the schools. Fluoridation is a topic that is controversial in some communities; a discussion, if it is properly conducted, may lead to a change of opinion. The establishing of clinical services for school children is another topic where the discussion method is valuable.

Questioning Method. No discussion can proceed without questioning. The proper use of questions is an important technique in itself. It can be very effective or it can be completely ineffective and disruptive. Spontaneous questions need to be controlled in large groups in order to conserve time. Antagonistic attitudes should not be tolerated, but different points of view, properly set forth, are essential to success in discussion. Classroom activities should be made natural and interesting with questions presented in a conversational tone. The teacher may address a rhetorical question to the group to start discussion. Rhetorical questions are usually prepared by the teacher or group leader before the discussion. They do not require an answer, but may state the purpose and aim of the discussion. One example is "Have you ever thought about why we have teeth?"

Developmental Method. The developmental or discovery method of teaching is used widely at present by teachers as a "new method." In reality it has been used for a long time in education. It is the "let's find out" approach used in the primary grades. It is a problem-solving technique in the upper grades. Children are taught to think through a problem and attempt solutions based on information gathered during some type of investigation. Dental health taught in this way is usually conducted by the classroom teacher. He may use resource personnel such as the dental hygienist to provide the basic facts upon which the investigation depends. Several periods are required for the project.

Example: What happens to teeth when sugars are allowed to remain on them? (rhetorical question) *Project:* Show how acid produced by fermentation of sugars causes decay of teeth. Class activities will require forming committees; reading pertinent books and articles; laboratory demonstration; library research for information and discussion of findings; and finally, writing the report.

Directed Study and Practice Method. Textbook study assigned and followed by recitation is still an essential part of learning by the individual. It may precede other types of classroom activities to form a base of reference or it may follow a classroom presentation to continue the motivation and interest in a problem. Since there is a quantity of literature produced by many sources on dental health, it is wise to use as much of it as possible to broaden the knowledge of proper control of dental disease and to emphasize the value of good dental health. Pamphlets, textbooks and magazine references provided after a lecture, demonstration or discussion on dental health tend to crystallize learning. Directed study is also an excellent form of review.

Team Teaching Method. We have heard a great deal since 1956 about team teaching. The United States Commission on Experimental Study and the Utilization of Staff in the Secondary School proposed and conducted experimental studies for improving teacher utilization in order to solve the teacher shortage. The major elements of team teaching are:

1. Two or more teachers working cooperatively with a certain group or groups of students on a specific subject matter.

2. Provisions for the team to work cooperatively in planning, instructing and evaluating the progress of students.

3. Flexible groupings, both large and small, to facilitate the use of time and appropriate methods of instruction.

4. A flexible daily schedule for group and individual students.

5. Provision for preparing and supplying

instructional media for large and small groups and for individual students.*

Team teaching can be adapted to dental health instruction with good results in school systems where specialized personnel is limited. In many schools dental hygienists are employed as resource people. They are required to service a large number of students in several schools. Team teaching, with the dental hygienist addressing large groups of students through closed circuit television or in auditorium assemblies followed by classroom visits and projects conducted by the classroom teachers using the dental hygienist as a consultant, is feasible and educationally sound. It requires special training of dental hygienists to prepare and present this type of instruction. The technique is best applied in secondary schools but may be adapted on a less elaborate scale to elementary levels from fourth to sixth grades and in junior high schools. The value of team teaching is in the use of specialized personnel to provide authentic information to large groups of students; providing information to classroom teachers; using visual aids and equipment economically and to the best advantage.

Lesson plans using the methods described here are presented in following chapters.

Questions for Review and Discussion

1. What is meant by "frame of reference" in dental health education?

2. Give reasons why unguided learning may be inadequate or misleading.

3. Based on the criteria applied to

* Adapted from Risk, T. M.: PRINCIPLES AND PRACTICES OF TEACHING IN SECONDARY SCHOOLS, American Book Company, New York, 4th Edition, 1968, p. 287.

methods of teaching, list each subject you are presently studying and indicate how the method employed does or does not fulfill the suggested criteria.

4. Choose the method of teaching you like best and explain why you like it and give an example of how an instructor made a subject interesting by using this method.

5. Suggest a number of dental health areas that could be used in the team teaching approach.

6. In the library find sources of illustrated materials that could be used in team teaching.

7. Conduct a discussion based on a controversial dental health problem with committees to do the initial investigation and a student team leader. Consider yourself as the teacher.

8. How would you cope with a group who tried to disrupt a discussion by asking impertinent questions?

9. Prepare a laboratory demonstration for some phase of dental health instruction other than toothbrushing.

10. Assume that you are a teacher who will lead a group discussion with high school students. What preliminary preparations should you make?

Selected Readings

Clark, H. L., Starr, I. S.: SECONDARY SCHOOL TEACHING METHODS, Part IV, The Macmillan Company, New York, 2nd Edition, 1967.

Pfeil, M. P.: "Off the Shelf and into the Classroom," American Education, U.S. Department of Health, Education and Welfare Office of Education. August-September, 1970, p. 13.

Risk, T. M.: PRINCIPLES AND PRACTICES OF TEACHING IN SECONDARY SCHOOLS, American Book Company, New York, 4th Edition, 1968.

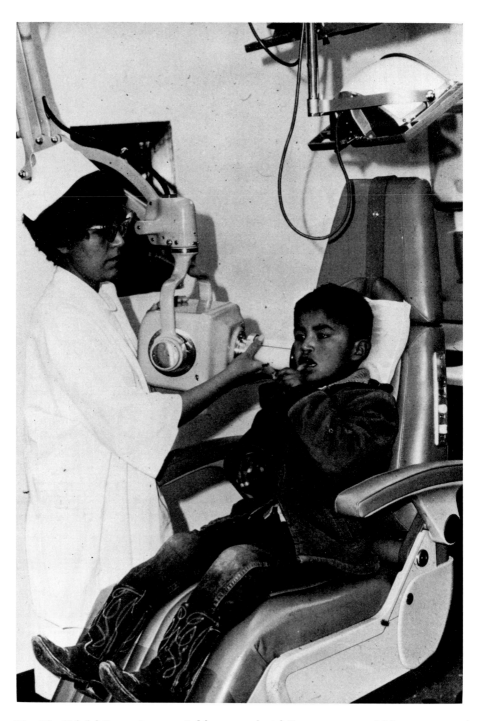

FIG. 25.—The Helpful Spy: A one-period lesson on dental X rays prepares children to accept them as part of dental treatment. (Courtesy, Indian Health Service, Dental Branch, U.S. Public Health Service, Department of Health, Education and Welfare.)

Chapter 13

Units of Teaching in Dental Health

The efforts of the dental health teacher should be focused on interpreting the principles of good dental health into meaningful learning experiences for the pupil. The purposes of dental health education go beyond emphasis on information into the development of daily dental health habits and attitudes. The specific techniques to achieve the best results should be carefully screened and constantly reviewed in the light of the following:

1. Only information that can be readily understood should be given at each grade level.

2. The amount of information should increase through the grades.

3. Factual information increases as the child develops the ability to understand and to recognize his own need for knowledge relating to dental health.

4. Instruction must be focused on the individual.

5. Learning experiences must be relevant to the need and the interest of the child.

6. Experience and instruction should provide a body of knowledge which will permit the child to make wise decisions.

7. Concepts should be developed through experiences so that transfer of learning from one situation to another takes place.

8. The facts and materials presented must be accurate and in accord with most recent scientific thought.

9. Dental health instruction should be based on activities that provide opportunities for good dental health practices.

10. Instruction should be based on the concept that controversial issues should be explored and that decisions reached should be on the basis of scientific judgement rather than on emotional bias.

11. Instruction in dental health should include sufficient understanding of scientific terms to provide the child with a vocabulary adequate for intelligent reading and understanding within his grade level.

12. Instruction in dental health should be developed as an independent unit of health education. Correlation with other areas of health education will have significance.

13. Instructional experiences in dental health should include opportunities for understanding and cooperating with the school, the home and the community.

Teaching Units are Organized

Units of teaching may be defined as the organization of topics and learning experiences in such a manner that they relate to a central theme or problem. Thus, it is important that objectives, the content, the teaching aids, the activities and the means of evaluation be written in a definite form to be followed by the teacher. Several types of unit organization follow in the text.

Direct dental health teaching requires definite planning.

121

A., Dental health education is concerned with everyday living.

B., Dental health education deals with specific facts.

C., Dental health education must be positive in its approach.

D., Dental health education attempts to improve the pupil's physical and mental health. It corrects misinformation; changes attitudes that adversely affect dental health; promotes good dental health practices and stimulates continuous interest in dental hygiene.

Steps in the Preparation of a Unit of Dental Health Instruction

Dental health guides and syllabi exist in almost every state. They are excellent guides for classroom teachers. They are prepared by experts in education assisted by members of the dental profession. Much of the teaching in dental health is based on these guides with the result that as they become dated, teachers run out of materials, children run out of interest and instruction tends to lose prestige in the curriculum. Only when dental health teaching is based on the interest and needs of each individual class does the subject matter remain interesting and challenging to the pupils. The educational policies of the school, the creative ability of the dental health teacher and the classroom teacher's cooperation will largely determine the content and the success of a dental health program of instruction.

In order to prevent stagnation and repetition, there are a number of principles which should guide the dental health educator. These are as follows:

1. Consider the entire plan of dental health instruction in terms of the range of classes to be taught.

2. Prepare a complete list of the dental health facts which the child should know when he completes his education.

3. Divide this list into areas of learning that seem to fit into the development and interests of children at certain age levels.

4. Prepare a list of materials that can be used as references.

5. Indicate the desired outcomes in habit formation for each area of learning.

Suggested Topics for Dental Health Instruction by Grades

The following brief outline provides topics for dental health instruction in each grade. The topics are chosen on the basis of group readiness, needs and interests.

Grade 1. Health teaching evolves around the child and the group in which he lives, namely the class.
Subjects to be taught:
1. Mouth hygiene and regular toothbrushing leading to regular habit formation.
2. Detergent foods versus sweets; finishing all the foods on our plates.
3. Awareness of teeth; the number of teeth in the primary set.
4. The dentist is a friend; a visit to the dentist; why teeth need fillings; dental care experiences.
5. Accident prevention in relation to teeth.

Grade 2. The child experiences his first accomplishment in school, progressing to the second grade. His dental health is also progressing. He loses first teeth and acquires new teeth.
Subjects to be taught:
1. Why do teeth fall out?
2. Sixth-year molars, their importance and care.
3. Why teeth decay and how they are repaired.
4. Special care at home through toothbrushing; review of method of toothbrushing.

Grade 3. Progress in body growth and development leads to interest in new teeth that are growing also.

Subjects to be taught:
1. Review toothbrushing technique.
2. Why do we use a dentifrice?
3. How to make a dentifrice.
4. What type of toothbrush should we use?
5. How does the dentist protect our teeth?
6. Why are regular visits to the dentist necessary?
7. Survey the class. What have we accomplished in dental health? What more do we need to do?

Grade 4. Interest centers in the functions and care of the body
Subjects to be taught:
1. The form and function of teeth.
2. Human teeth compared to animal teeth.
3. What happens when a tooth is lost?
4. Foods for chewing exercise.
5. Review how we care for our teeth.

Grade 5. Children have good appetites at this age and interest in food is high.
Subjects to be taught:
1. Study of basic food requirements.
2. Study of food groups.
3. Harmful effects of foods containing free sugars in reference to dental health.
4. Proper use and control of food high in sugars.
5. The function of vitamins in nutrition.
6. Natural sources of vitamins.
7. Control of artificial vitamin intake.
8. Function of minerals in the diet.
9. Phosphorus and calcium in tooth development.

10. The effects of poor nutrition and inadequate diet on the health of the teeth.
11. Correcting deficiencies by improved food habits.
12. Study of food habits and dental health in the countries studied in social studies course.

Grade 6. Concentration is on accident prevention and good health practices.
Subjects to be taught:
1. Review of home care and regular dental health services.
2. General review of calcium and phosphorus in building sound teeth.
3. Accident prevention in competitive games, with special reference to teeth.
4. What to do in case of accidents to teeth.
5. The effects of neglect of teeth after accidents.
6. Discussion of malocclusion.
7. Consumer education on dentifrices and toothbrushes.
8. Detailed study of tooth structures.

In schools consisting of all eight grades the following subjects may be taught. Normally these are given in junior high school.

Grade 7. Body growth and development in reference to athletic ability are of great interest.
Subjects to be taught:
A project on tooth development in terms of form, structure and function should be developed, including the following broad areas:
1. Detailed study of teeth including hard and soft structures in the mouth.
2. The action and function of chewing.
3. The effect of tooth loss on

speech, face and head development and appearance.

4. Correction of tooth loss by adequate dental care.
5. Effective correction of malocclusion; cooperation during treatment; long-term advantages.
6. Teeth as a source of infection. Herpes and group infections; caries as individual infection; systemic infection related to the tissues surrounding teeth.

Grade 8. Children graduating from grade school are faced with a period of complete change either into high schools or vocational education including possible part-time employment. It is important to stress the effects of dental neglect and the responsibility of the individual for his own health.

Subjects to be taught:

1. Review the process of dental decay.
2. Advantages of prevention: financial, personal appearance; methods of prevention.
3. Use of the X ray in dental diagnosis.
4. Research findings in reference to dental disease.
5. Personal responsibility for continuous dental care.
6. Community responsibilities for dental care of indigents.
7. Use of the class dental inspection to evaluate the dental health of the group in terms of:
   a. How much has been done to prevent dental disease?
   b. What has been accomplished in increasing motivation and habit formation for personal dental hygiene?
   c. What are the further

needs of the group?
   d. How can individuals meet their dental needs?

Grades 9 through 12. Senior high school. The period of puberty creates a series of emotional problems that can wreck the health of boys and girls. They are neglectful of their diet, resorting to foods with high sugar content for quick energy. They are over-active and consider adquate sleep unimportant. These excesses bring on two aspects of dental disease: (1) an increase in caries susceptibility and (2) the onset of periodontal disease. Because they are being taught their duties and obligations as citizens, water fluoridation is a good topic to encourage them in community activity.

Subjects to be taught:

1. A scientific study of nutrition as it relates to the diet of the adolescent, correlating with information about the use of tobacco, alcohol and drugs.
2. A review of caries control methods.
3. Public acceptance of fluoridation of the communal water supply including: the history, the effectiveness, costs, pros and cons of fluoridation, professional organization acceptance of and participation in the local community program for fluoridation.
4. A study of the causes and effects of periodontal disease as it pertains to the onset of the disease during adolescence and the effects on health in adult life.
5. The teeth and supporting tissues as indicators of health status.
6. Careers in dentistry, includ-

ing the dental team: dentist, dental hygienist, dental assistant, dental technician.

Topics for Discussion According to Class Needs

1. Toothbrushing: the toothbrush, selection, use and care; dentifrices, facts and fallacies; cleanliness a social asset; forming desirable dental health habits.
2. Why do we have two sets of teeth? Primary teeth, the sixth-year molars, permanent teeth. Why teeth are "shed." Why teeth should last as long as life. Do animals have more than one set? What happens when teeth wear down? How can we prevent loss of teeth?
3. The dentist and his contribution to dental health; dental X rays, filling teeth, replacing teeth, periodic cleaning of teeth, regular dental appointments, release time from school for dental appointments. What can be learned in a dental office?
4. Why do we have a dental inspection in school? What is individual dental health appraisal? What are the problems of dental health in the home, the school and the community?
5. The structure, development and functions of teeth; teeth in relation to digestion; relation of occlusion to efficient mastication and appearance; the consequences of losing a permanent tooth.
6. Enemies of dental health; process of tooth decay, fractured teeth, stains and deposits on teeth, malocclusion, the health of the supporting structures of the teeth; undesirable habits.
7. Methods of prevention; early and regular dental care; topical application of stannous fluoride, addition of fluorides to communal water supplies; avenues of prevention being explored in research.
8. The effects of dental neglect; why people do not obtain dental care; cost of early treatment versus cost of neglect.
9. Diet in relation to good teeth and good health; the school lunch, healthful snacks, effects of sugars; mouth cleanliness as a factor of diet control; food elements that contribute to dental health.

For junior and senior high school the following broad topics are suggested after the basic understanding of the above-mentioned topics have been explored.

1. Dental Health Quiz: what do we know about ourselves? Review of dental health knowledge, correct fallacies, re-establish dental health facts.
2. Responsibilities of the individual, the family, the school and the community for the dental health of children.
3. Community needs in relation to dental health; community resources that attempt to meet these needs; action needed for establishing better facilities for dental health.
4. Dental Research: implications for the present and for the future; consumer education in relation to purchasing dental services, toothbrushes and dentifrices; changing concepts in dental health procedures; effects of dental health on economic and social success.

Suggested Activities for Dental Health Education

Primary and Intermediate Elementary Grades

Bulletin Boards

Display a collection of magazine pictures brought to school by the children.
Display a series of pamphlets on dental health.
Pin up stories written by the children about their dental experiences.
Display a series of posters (one at a time) on a rotating basis.

Demonstrations

Use a large brush and tooth model to demonstrate proper method of toothbrushing. Have the children practice the strokes by using the index finger as a brush on the outside of the cheek.

Make a simple tooth powder of salt, bicarbonate of soda and a few drops of peppermint. Have small envelope filled with the powder to take home.

Illustrate acid in the mouth by placing litmus paper on the tongue. Let each child test his mouth. Place a piece of litmus paper in a glass of water and note the color, then place litmus paper in a solution of vinegar and water and note the change of color. Explain the concept of pH.

Prepare a snack party of raw vegetables and fruit or nuts instead of foods with large amounts of sugar.

Give each child a disclosing wafer to chew and let him observe the plaque on his own teeth.

Have children rinse their mouth with water after lunch, catch the rinse in a paper cup and observe the food debris. Rinse several times, then catch the last rinse in the cup and note how food debris has been rinsed away.

Check Lists

After the dental inspection in school, prepare a class list in checklist form indicating missing teeth, filled teeth, decayed teeth and patterns of toothbrushing. Record each child on the list but *do not use names*. Let each child play "Guess Who" and locate his own record on the list.

Prepare a mimeographed sheet to be taken home which indicates when the teeth are brushed, with spaces for morning, after breakfast, after lunch, after dinner and at bedtime. Have the sheets rated by the teacher after one week.

Prepare a checklist of dental experiences for each child to be kept for one semester in school to show dental health efforts. Include:

	Date	Date
I had my teeth examined.		
I had X rays taken.		
I had dental work completed.		
I had fluoride treatments.		
My dentist recommends that I return.		

Prepare a diet checklist. This list should contain the requirements of a good diet for breakfast, lunch, dinner and afternoon snacks. Leave space to check each meal during one week. The lists should be returned to school and discussed, with each child allowed to evaluate his own.

Discussions

Discuss the use of dentifrices and mouthwashes. Use ads to demonstrate.

Discuss the effects of premature loss of primary teeth on permanent teeth.

Show "smiling picture" and talk about how teeth add to appearance. Then blacken several teeth on the picture and let the children laugh.

Discuss foods and attitudes at meal time. Explain detergent foods. Show how sweet foods can be used as part of a meal.

Discuss tooth decay, how, why and when it happens.

Dramatizations

Set up a "pretend dental office" in a classroom and bring instruments to be used for examination. Let children take parts in discussing the use of the instruments. Let the "dentist" explain why he takes X rays. Have the "patient" ask questions. Let the "dental hygienist" explain what she does.

Children can write a play about accidents on the playground, show how to avoid them and what to do in case of an accident to teeth.

Have a sing-in by changing some of the words of known songs so that they apply to dental health.

Have a brush-in by using a fluoridated toothpaste. Supply brushes, paste and two paper cups, one with water.

Drawings

Have children copy and label a tooth from a chalkboard drawing. Write at the bottom of the picture what each part of the tooth does.

Let children use free expression by drawing in their chosen medium impressions of their first visit to the dentist or to the dental health office in school.

Have children express in free form and color their feelings about brushing their teeth.

Have children draw pictures of common articles which should not be put in the mouth. Then have them draw a toothbrush on the same sheet.

Exhibits

Prepare an exhibit of various types of toothbrushes, with an evaluation of each on a card.

Prepare a display of animal teeth and compare them with *models* of human teeth as to size, shape and function.

Show the process of decay with plaster models.

Make an exhibit of dental X rays by using mock-up or actual photographs of films, the x-ray machine and a child in a dental chair having X rays taken.

Prepare a "sugar tree" from a leafless branch, hang foods high in sugar content on it labeled with the amount of sugar in each food.

Make a flip chart showing the several parts of a tooth and ending with a completed tooth.

Make a flip chart of the four basic foods and the amounts of them required for good general health.

Make a flip chart of the process of decay.

Obtain plaster models of various types

of malocclusions and second models showing their corrections.

Show and Tell—Primary or Kindergarten

Children share experiences in the dental office, bring in cotton rolls and prizes given to them by the dentist.

Using puppets of the dentist, the dental hygienist and child, let the children improvise a visit to the dentist.

Junior and Senior High School

(In addition to those that may be adapted from the elementary school lists)

Interviews

Form a committee to interview the chief dental officer of an armed forces installation, a community clinic or a ghetto health center. Obtain information about the immediate problems of dental health and how the different groups are attempting to solve them. If more than one committee is interviewing, a discussion of the different problems should follow.

Interview the representative of the state health department, division of dental health and learn how the dental health program serves large numbers of people.

Interview a local dentist and ask what he thinks the most pressing needs of adolescents in relation to dental health are.

Interview two local citizens, one who advocates fluoridation of water supplies and one who opposes it. Compare their arguments.

All interviews should be written and reported to the class, then opened for discussion.

Debates

Because there is opposition in some communities, the most obvious debatable subject at present is, Should this community fluoridate its water supply?

Will free clinics jeopardize the private practice of the local dentist?

What are the effects of brush-ins that permit students to apply fluorides to their own teeth?

Panels

Arrange a panel of experts interested in the community dental problems. Include a local dentist, a public health official, a member of a minority group, a health educator and a student. Let the panel choose the subject. "The school dental health program leaves something to be desired." A student panel can discuss this subject, and suggest changes that will make the program more effective and interesting to adolescents.

Arrange a panel for the discussion of the use of alcohol, tobacco and drugs in reference to dental health. Have a local dentist act as moderator.

Self-evaluation Tests

Provide each student with a list of true-false questions that will indicate his attitudes and habits regarding dental health. Compare his answers with the best information on good dental health routines.

Students may keep track of food intake for a period of one week, indicating each day his consumption in a plus or minus column under the four basic foods and the quantity required for an adequate diet.

Encourage students to evaluate their scholastic aptitude for careers in dentistry, as a dentist, as a dental hygienist, as a dental assistant or a laboratory technician. Give professional evaluation when a student asks.

Field Trips

Visit the fluoridation plant in the local water district. How many people are served by it? What is the approximate cost per 1,000 people?

Visit a preschool facility in a ghetto neighborhood. What is being done to educate parents to the dental needs of children? Who is responsible for dental treatment? What community facilities are available for treatment of very young children?

Visit a home for the disabled. What are their problems in dental health? How do they differ from those of normal individuals? How are the dental programs financed?

Charts

Chart the dental health status of the individuals of a class at the beginning of the school year. Include the following: lost permanent teeth, filled permanent teeth, periodontal conditions, mouth hygiene and tooth replacement. Compare this chart with a similar one at the end of the year. Document the improvement. Compare with national averages.

The unit of work provided here as an example of a written plan is suitable for the junior high school level. Educators agree that a specific unit of dental health instruction at this age level, twelve to fifteen years of age, is advisable for the following reasons:

1. Through the elementary grades dental health experiences may be only in terms of incidental teaching as the growth and development of body and mind proceed.

2. The areas of dental health instruction have grown out of the needs of the individual and the group at each grade level.

3. There appears to be a need for a general drawing together of all the dental health experiences into a positive approach to dental health. This objective may be met by providing specific facts and experiences that will serve the individual throughout the life span.

4. Since many children do not proceed to senior high school, the junior high school level reaches the greatest number of children during the adolescent period.

Table 8. *Your Teeth—For Life*

Group:	Junior high school, 12 to 15 years of age.
Time Required:	Five to six weeks
Approximate Number of Classes:	Ten to fifteen
Periods:	Forty minutes each

Objectives:
1. To provide basic scientific knowledge so that pupils will know and understand reasons for preserving their teeth in a healthy condition during the entire life span.
2. To provide motivation for good dental health practices.
3. To stimulate interest in the problems of dental health from the personal, the family and the community point of view.

Basic knowledge to be learned:
1. The structure and function of teeth.
2. The care of the teeth, including personal efforts and services provided by the dentist. Causes and control of dental diseases.
3. The realization of dental health as a community problem and the individual's responsibility in solving it.
4. Although dental health is obtainable, many people fail to secure the services needed for good teeth.

Initiating the unit:
1. Period of questions and answers by pupils and teacher.
2. Prepare class for the showing of the film, "Matter of Choice" (DH51) (American Dental Association).
   Observe in the film: The services of the dentist, the process of decay, the effect of good teeth on you as a viewer.
3. Show the film and follow with an evaluation of it.
   Class questions arising from the film; points to recall through questions by the teacher. Activity: pupils write a short critique of the film.
4. Assignment: Use text available in library.

5. Discuss the text, answer questions.
6. Class discussion on possible activities and projects, selection of committees, sources of information, recording and reporting.

Suggested activities:
1. Group I. To obtain three dimensional models of teeth, illustrations of teeth and their supporting tissues; make a chart of the substances that are found in teeth (mineral and organic); arrange materials as a display in the classroom.
2. Group II. Provide a speaker for the demonstration of the American Dental Association recommended toothbrushing technique. Provide illustrations and pictures. Conduct the meeting to which the speaker will be invited.
3. Group III. Prepare illustrations of the processes of tooth decay; evaluate the dental health of the class by preparing a graph of the incidence of dental decay as disclosed by the dental health records of the school. Prepare a list of sources for dental treatment in the community. Discuss this report in class.
4. Group IV. Write and present a report on the known methods of preventing dental decay; include information from magazines, radio and television. Conduct a discussion period in class on the selection of a toothbrush, evaluation of advertising of dentifrices and mouthwashes.
5. Group V. Assemble sources of information used by Groups I to IV. Prepare a bibliography for class distribution. Write a brief narration of the class activities.

Methods of evaluation:

1. Provide a period of review of the subject matter covered.
2. Give a final test, including objective questions and essay questions, to evaluate individual achievement.

3. Have the dental hygiene teacher conduct a class inspection for toothbrushing habits and dental corrections. Read and evaluate the report of the inspection.
4. Evaluate pupils on the basis of partici-

Table 9. *Dental Health Unit—High School: Look at Your Periodontium*

Concepts: More teeth are lost in adult life through breakdown of the periodontium than through dental decay. The health of the gingiva and bony support of the teeth depend to a large measure on excellent mouth hygiene. Periodontal disease is preventable and curable. Diet affects mouth health.

Objectives and Goals	Activities	Materials and Resources

Action Learning
Practices good mouth hygiene
Visits the dentist or dental hygienist for routine prophylaxis, X rays, observation
Maintains a good diet for good health
Establishes a healthful routine of exercise, recreation and personal hygiene
Refrains from use of alcohol, tobacco and drugs
 	
Affective Learning
Realizes the value of good mouth hygiene—physically, mentally and socially
Realizes the value of health supporting tissues in maintaining teeth for a lifetime
Knows that periodontal disease is preventable and curable
Understands the function of the various tissues surrounding the teeth
 	
Cognitive Learning
Demonstrates interest in mouth health by self-evaluation
Realizes that alcohol, tobacco and drugs are dangerous to dental health
Accepts dental health as part of the process of growing to adulthood
Knows the results of dental neglect
Understands the relationship of nutrition to periodontal health
	Demonstrations
	Prepare an exhibit of one tooth with healthy supporting tissues and one showing gingival inflammation
	Prepare a series of Petri plates showing types of bacteria involved in gingivitis
	Prepare a series of X rays showing the breakdown of periodontal support
	
	Discussion
	Define dental terms
	Periodontal disease is a worldwide problem
	Conditions that lead to various types of periodontal diseases
	What effect do drugs, alcohol and tobacco have on these tissues?
	What is the effect of malnutrition?
	What constitutes a good diet?
	
	Displays
	In the library
	  Posters on good diet
	  Dental health units
	    in text books
	  Current articles in periodicals
	    relating to dental health
	American Dental Association
	  Exhibit and literature on
	    "There is Nothing Abstract About Smoking"
	Hall bulletin boards
	  materials on good diet from
	    National Dairy Council
	    (111 North Canal St.
	    Chicago, Ill.)
		"Beware of Plaque, It Causes Tooth Loss," U. S. Public Health poster
		From the biology department collect materials for bacterial display
		"Your Guide to Oral Health" obtain copies for each student, American Dental Association
		Film Strips
		  "Periodontics"
		  "Good Brushing Technique"
		  Professional Research Inc.
		  461 N. Lea Brea Ave.
		  Los Angeles, Calif. 90036
		"How Can We Teach Adolescents about Smoking, Drinking and Drug Abuse?" Reprint, Journal of Health and Physical Education, October, 1968, National Education Association
		"Elements of an Effective Program of Dental Health for Children." Journal of School Health, October, 1970.
		"Periodontics"
		  Dental Science Handbook
		  American Dental Association

Time requirement   Forty-five minute period each day for one week.
Conference of health educator and dental hygiene teacher.

pation in group activities, special reports, results of objective achievement test and dental health achievement.

Dental Health Instruction for High School Students

Teen-agers have a higher incidence of dental decay than any other group of school children. They also show a lack of mouth hygiene. Periodontal disease may have taken toll of the supporting tissues and the general health of the mouth and teeth suffer from poor nutrition. It is a challenge to interest these students in dental health, for most of them have been exposed to some degree of dental health instruction during their elementary schooling. The problem is

---

Table 10.   The Helpful Spy*

One Period Study of Dental X Rays for Intermediate Elementary Grades:

Objectives:
> To discover what an X ray is
> To learn why dental X rays are needed before dental treatment
> To remove fear of x-ray exposure
> To explain precautions against excess radiation

Materials:
> Mock-up illustration of tooth forms covered with gingiva
> Mock-up illustration of tooth forms as seen in an X ray
> Shadow box with actual X ray showing cavities between teeth
> Blank film packets and exposed films to be handled by children
> Mock-up or actual illustration of dental x-ray machine

Statement:
> This is the actual wording of the lecture which is divided into three parts

Introduction
> Short history of the discovery of X rays
> The value of X rays in dental treatment

Procedure
> Give a clear account of the technique of exposing and processing dental films
> Compare this procedure with pictures taken by a camera
> Question pupils about their experiences with dental X rays
> Explain the precautions that the dentist takes in exposing films
> Clarify any misconceptions about over-exposure
> Prepare children for the experience of having X rays taken during dental treatment by dispelling fear of the machine, the actual exposure and the discomfort of holding the film in the mouth

Evaluation:
> Did the class show interest in the materials used?
> Did they respond with questions to your talk?
> Were you sure of yourself in answering questions and using visual aids?

---

*Adapted from the pamphlet of the American Dental Association

to stimulate high school students so as to arouse interest in a subject that seems far from their daily needs and "childish" in its content.

Safety Education: Implications for Dental Health

It is not difficult to discover why safety education has become an important part of the curriculum in all grades. Accidents cause the death of 95,000 persons each year. There are 9,500,000 non-fatal accidents and injuries each year. The National Safety Council estimates that accidents cost the American people approximately 12 billion dollars annually. Safety education teaches children to avoid accidents by knowing the hazards and avoiding risks. The following areas of safety instruction in school have dental implications.

KINDERGARTEN (CHILDREN FIVE YEARS OLD)
Living Together
  Proper use and handling of equipment
  Proper method of walking up and down stairs
  Proper use of the swings on the playground

Dental Health Teaching
  Avoid putting foreign objects in the mouth; biting on pencils, etc.
  Falls cause broken front teeth and fractured jaws
  A child may have several teeth knocked out by a swing

GRADES 1 TO 3 (CHILDREN SIX TO EIGHT YEARS OLD)
Health Needs and Interests Related to Growth Period
  Exercise and play with abundance of energy
  Bicycling and climbing. New skills in skating

Dental Health Teaching
  Head-on collisions result in injury to lips and possible chipping of upper anterior teeth.

Report any mouth injury due to "spills" immediately to the health room. Teeth may be saved by quick action and treatment.

GRADES 4 TO 6 (STUDENTS NINE TO ELEVEN YEARS OLD)
How to Plan the Daily Program So as to Allow Ample Time for Schoolwork, Play and Rest.
  Take time for health practices
  Recognize health and safety hazards
  Prepare a checklist of safety hazards in the home
  Watch for undesirable habits
  Toothbrushing immediately after eating prevents tooth decay.
  Drinking fountains may be hazardous to teeth unless pushing and shoving are avoided while children drink.
  Among these mention running with sharp or pointed objects in the mouth; chipping teeth by biting on too-hard objects. Nail biting; thumb and finger sucking; tongue thrusting; undue chewing habits; grinding the teeth under strain.

JUNIOR HIGH SCHOOL (STUDENTS ELEVEN TO FOURTEEN YEARS OLD)
  Accidents reach their peak during this period. There is marked increase in school accidents in shops, gymnasiums and stairways
  Again emphasize the need for immediate attention in case of accidents to teeth. Use tools with care so that one's neighbor will not be injured, especially around the face and mouth. Permanent teeth must be protected to last a lifetime.

SENIOR HIGH SCHOOL (STUDENTS FOURTEEN TO EIGHTEEN YEARS OLD)
  Main hazards are found in competitive sports and driving cars, motorcycles, scooters and other high-speed vehicles. The use of mouth protectors made of soft rubber or plastics prevents sudden shock to teeth. Encourage school regulations that require mouth and face pro-

tectors and enforce them. Encourage dental health projects in science fairs showing how accidents to mouth and teeth can be avoided.

Evaluating Pupil Achievement

Evaluation is the process by which the advancement in attaining the objectives of the unit is measured. Several reasons may be stated for including evaluation as a part of unit planning.

1. Evaluation helps the dental health educator to know where to place the emphasis in teaching the unit. It strengthens the weak areas of teaching.
2. Evaluation which the students conduct helps them to find out what prog-

ress they are making in health habits. It becomes an instrument of motivation.

3. When systematic instruction is given, evaluation may be used as a measure of learning dental health facts and of grading individual students.
4. Evaluation helps health councils and other groups in curriculum planning in relation to content and method.
5. The interest of school administrators can be increased in the overall dental health program if evaluation of teaching is properly and interestingly presented. It helps to "sell" the dental health program since administrators are accustomed to judging the efficiency of other areas of instruction by evaluation techniques.

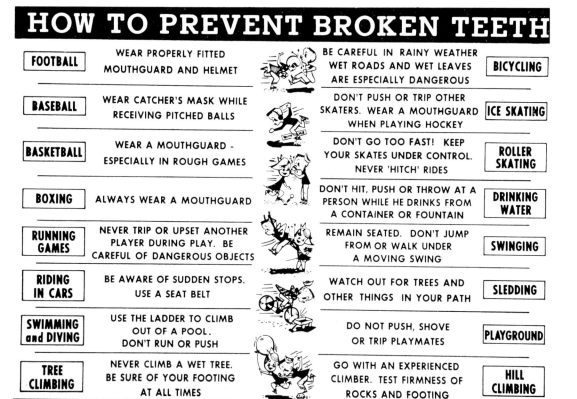

FIG. 26.

Table 11.   Dental Health Unit—Grade 3

Concepts: Body growth and development include newly erupted teeth. Regular daily home care protects teeth. Regular dental visits prevent pain and loss of permanent teeth. Safe play prevents dental accidents.

Objectives and Goals	Activities	Materials
Action Learning Brushes teeth after eating Visits the dentist regularly Acts safely to protect teeth *Affective Learning* Realizes the importance of regular toothbrushing Appreciates the importance of regular dental treatment Realizes that first teeth are shed and permanent teeth replace them Realizes that permanent teeth must last a lifetime Uses school equipment safely *Cognitive Learning* Can demonstrate proper toothbrushing technique Knows why dentifrice is used Comprehends the function of teeth and their relation to good general health Knows accident hazards to teeth	*Demonstrations* Make a dentifrice powder and paste. After lunch or snack chew a disclosing tablet to show plaque and debris. Brush and reapply disclosing tablet to show where toothbrush failed to clean the teeth. *Discussion* The dentist is a friend. Why do we have two sets of teeth? What do teeth do for appearance, for health, for social adjustment? Why do we have a dental health week? How safe is our classroom? *Display* Prepare a bulletin board of dentifrice ads with comments. Using a shadow box show X rays of jaws with primary and permanent teeth Display colorful booklets and health texts from the library	Large toothbrush and tooth models Film or film strip on dental health from school library Obtain a supply of a pamphlet on dental hygiene to be taken home Bring library books on dental health and safety to the classroom to be used in free reading time Obtain soda and salt, small paper mixing cups and small envelopes for taking dentifrice home Model of a primary tooth Model of a permanent tooth Word list of dental terms for the teacher

Time Schedule
School dental hygienist has conference with teacher before initiating the unit.
Hygienist sets up displays, demonstrations and library materials.
Hygienist gives two 25-minute talks one week apart.
Teacher checks for brushed teeth 15 minutes each morning during the week between talks.
Teachers answers questions on dental health, reviews new learnings and teaches new word list.

Evaluation of a dental health unit should take into consideration: a, how much has been learned from the facts presented; b, what changes in attitudes and behavior have resulted.

Questions for Review and Discussion

1. Test your understanding of educational concepts as they apply to dental health instruction. Mark the following statements true(T) or false(F). Consider the full statement before making a decision.

_____ A. It is good teaching to repeat certain information, but as the child progresses from grade to grade the detail and approach should change.

_____ B. Dental health can be effectively taught as incidental teaching in all grades.

_____ C. The time to teach about the sixth-year molar is in the sixth grade when most of the second teeth have erupted.

_____ D. Children should be taught to accept the inconvenience and at times the discomfort of dental treatment as a means of maintaining good dental health.

_____ E. If a child has good teeth and appears to be free of dental disease, he need not be concerned with the factual instruction in dental health.

_____ F. Children must be motivated to bridge the gap between dental health instruction and habit formation.

_____ G. Change can take place in habits and knowledge concerning dental health through participation in a complete dental health education program.

_____ H. The dental health program needs to be evaluated constantly to be sure that teachers and children are aware of changes in dental health that result from research.

_____ I. Although simple terms are used in place of scientific words, children need to build a considerable vocabulary of dental terms in order to understand dental health facts.

_____ J. Activity programs do not apply in dental health instruction since the school environment is not conducive to such activities as brushing the teeth after the school lunch.

2. Accidents to teeth in school are numerous. Make a survey of a classroom or a home and enumerate the number of hazards that were found. Discuss the findings in class.

3. Make a list of dental health projects that might be used in a school science fair.

4. Write a short dramatization that will help to dispel fear of dental treatment.

5. Write out the preparation for a single lecture on dental health. Use your own judgment as to the subject.

6. Write the lecture material for the lesson plan, "Look at Your Periodontium."

7. It has been said that instruction should be focused upon the individual and his needs. Name four ways of discovering these needs.

8. Explain how dental health education is concerned with everyday living.

9. Write a lesson plan for the first grade.

10. What would you say to a class of small children to inspire them to *draw* their impressions of a visit to the dentist?

Selected Readings

Articles

"A Position on School Dental Health Education," Journal of School Health, September, 1970, p. 361.

"Development and Testing of a Junior High School Oral Hygiene Education Program," Journal of School Health, December, 1970, p. 557.

"Elements of an Effective Program of Dental Health for School Age Children," Journal of School Health, October, 1970, p. 421.

"New Forms of Dental Health Education," Journal Public Health Dentistry, Fall Issue, 1970, p. 218.

"Oral Hygiene Performance of Elementary School Children Following Dental Health Education," Journal of Dentistry for Children, July-August, 1970, p. 298.

"The Dental Hygienist and Better Oral Health for School Children," Journal of The Academy of General Dentistry, January, 1971.

"The Oral Hygiene of High School Students as Affected by Three Different Educational Programs," Journal Public Health Dentistry, Spring Issue, 1967, p. 91.

Texts and Pamphlets

DENTAL SCIENCE HANDBOOK, American Dental Association and the National Institute of Dental Research, 1970. Chicago, Ill.

Fletcher, C. M., Horn, D. (WHO Consultants): "Smoking and Health," U.S. Department of Health, Education and Welfare, National Communicable Disease Center, Atlanta, Georgia, 1970.

Graded Series of Health Texts, California State Department of Education, Sacramento, California, 1967.

Stoll, F. A., Catherman, J. L.: DENTAL HEALTH EDUCATION, Chapter 11 (Extensive reference lists), Lea & Febiger, Philadelphia, 3rd Edition, 1967.

PART IV

THE ROLE OF INSTRUCTIONAL MATERIALS IN DENTAL HEALTH EDUCATION

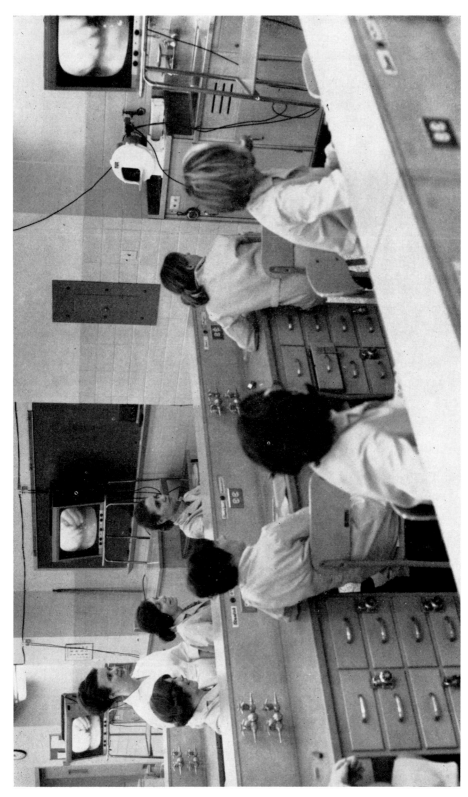

Fig. 27.—Closed circuit television permits several classes to tune in to one lecture or demonstration, thus conserving the time of the special teachers. It is used in team teaching. (Courtesy, Department of Dental Hygiene, School of Dentistry, Marquette University.)

Chapter 14

Educational Media and Learning Opportunities

Audiovisual Devices

Audiovisual devices are used as methods of building concepts. They are not meant to take the place of the teacher or to assume the actual task of teaching. Visual aids are open to serious abuses, however. In order to be effective in the learning process, the purpose of the visual aid must be clearly explained to the learner. If he merely becomes a viewer instead of a doer, thought has been removed from the situation. Unless he forms a critical attitude and cultivates good judgment while viewing he does not benefit from the use of the visual aid.

If audiovisual aids are properly used they contribute to the formation of desirable concepts, provide interest for abstract ideas and tend to make learning permanent. Dental health touches on every phase of living and every medium of communication. Recognition of the importance of dental health is found in the quantity and quality of source material available for teaching. Materials must contribute directly to the purpose of the program. Some of these materials are: books, pamphlets and periodicals, bulletin boards, films, film strips and slides, flannel boards, pictures, records or tape recordings and television.

There is another group of learning experiences known as group or individual interactions. These include buzz sessions or small group discussions, field trips, class discussions, lectures, panel discussions, role playing or sociodrama and symposiums. These educational media will be discussed in the next chapter.

Instructional material selected for a particular unit must be based on criteria of learning and meet the objectives and goals of the unit. Is it motivating? Is it interesting? Is it a rewarding experience? Does it contribute to change of habits and attitudes? Does it make learning of information permanent?

As students progress they mature and their learning experiences should become more complex. They are capable of learning information that may not directly concern their immediate needs.

Elements to consider in selecting materials for instruction are:

1. Is the material presented at an opportune time? Tired students do not observe, listen or learn well.

2. The class size will affect the selection of materials and media. Sometimes it is good teaching to divide large classes into smaller groups to facilitate informal discussion. Films, film strips and television can be shown effectively to large groups.

3. Time allotment is crucial in the busy school day. Plan experiments, films and group activities within the time allotted. Do not infringe upon time set for other activities.

4. Be sure that the equipment needed is available. Order it ahead of time and

become acquainted with the operation of the different types of projectors and other aids. Review the film before showing it.

5. All educational media are more effective when they are used in a good environment. Good lighting, seating so that all can see, good ventilation and proper room temperature are essential.

Chalk Boards

Definite skill and some artistic talent are required to use a chalk board (commonly known as a blackboard) for illustrating. It is better to use other visual aids such as pictures, posters or opaque projectors unless the dental health teacher has practiced freehand drawing. The chalk board is used primarily to show symbols, words and numbers. When writing on the blackboard be sure that all learners can see the board. Use the form of writing that is used by the classroom teacher. Printing is used in lower grades, script writing in upper grades. Dental health teachers should not use large areas of a chalk board and expect the material to remain there for a long time. The class teacher may need to use the chalk board. Avoid putting too much on the board at one time; it is confusing. Never stand directly in front of what is being written. Clean the board after the lesson unless the class teacher requests that it be left for further discussion.

Flannel Boards and Perforated Hard Boards

Flannel boards (a hard board covered with flannel or velvet) are used during lectures since materials can be placed, removed and rearranged at will. It is convenient to use; easily transported; takes little space and all the materials can be prepared ahead of time. Pictures and illustrations must be backed with coarse sandpaper in order for them to stick to the flannel board.

Perforated hard boards are good for semipermanent exhibits. Their value lies in the use of actual materials such as tooth forms, toothbrushes and tubes of dentifrice.

There are a number of ways to fasten materials to these peg boards.

Picture Study

Still pictures produced in color are abundant and easy to find. The values of dental health have been illustrated in many interesting ways by professional organizations and commercial companies. Caution is the word in selecting pictures to make sure that they are not biased and do not advertise a particular product. The principal value of pictures is to stimulate interest in collecting and discussing them. They help students to visualize what is being taught.

Posters, Bulletin Boards and Exhibits

Posters from many sources are obtainable free of charge or for a small price. They are important as visual materials in teaching dental health. They are seen in advertisements in window displays, car cards and billboards. We cannot avoid them and they have a strong influence on the public. Government agencies and health associations make use of them. Posters produced outside the school should be selected carefully if they are to be used in school.

Posters are used to motivate: Brush your teeth, Go to the dentist, Eat nourishing food. The poster emphasizes one idea. In choosing posters consider these points.

1. Is the message clear and concise, so that only a glance is needed to "get it across"?

2. Is the color pleasing and in proper contrast so that the observer will take a second glance?

3. Is the illustration attractive and pertinent?

4. Is the lettering easy to read?

5. Is the poster printed on suitable stock for display on several occasions?

If posters are made by children they should not be considered "art work" but rather an expression of how he feels about dental health and how he wants to express his feelings to others. Art teachers object to making posters and should not be asked to use their time for this purpose. However, they may be consulted about poster making and asked to supply the materials. The fact that a child can make a good poster does not necessarily indicate that he is convinced that *he* should practice good dental health habits. Poster contests are not held for the purpose of increasing motivation for better dental health, but rather, for the winning of a prize and supplying posters for others to use. Often the winners have poor dental health.

Bulletin boards are more complicated than posters. Several ideas may be conveyed by the bulletin board at one time. It may be displayed for a longer period of time in order to be seen by all learners but not so long that it becomes "old stuff." The main purpose of a bulletin board or an exhibit is to produce the effect of a pleasant shock that makes the learner want to stop, look and learn. A bulletin board can be a class project, with materials supplied by the pupils from library research, from the home or from the community. Such a bulletin board might be a map showing the dental offices and clinics within the community.

No dental health room should be without a bulletin board. It should be kept up-to-date with interesting new ideas and new materials. If properly used, it can be a good motivational force for increasing interest in dental health. The power of suggestion is a strong one. Exhibits and bulletin boards use it to advantage.

Motion Pictures, Slides, Film Strips and Television

These materials and media are grouped together because they are known as "passive materials" in their effect on the learners. Participation in the activity shown in the film is not required. They should be used as a teaching device rather than as a means of amusement in dental health instruction. The main value of films is that they provide realism and motion. They can display complicated situations step by step. The learner can see in a few moments what might have taken a long time to produce. Microorganisms that cannot be seen by the human eye become visible when seen under a high-powered microscope.

It is important that the dental health educator be thoroughly familiar with a film before the showing so that he may answer questions intelligently. It is well to prepare students for what they are about to see; to explain what they should look for and to orient them toward the message of the film. It is also a good plan to evaluate a film by testing learners on the main points that have been observed.

Types of Projectors

There are already a number of different types of projectors and new ones are appearing almost daily.

The Opaque Projector. This can show anything from a model of a tooth to a full written page, in actual color. No slides, transparencies or films are needed. This projector is excellent for use in both grade and high school because it can use materials that are available in the library, the laboratory and a number of other sources. It requires no special installation or wiring.

The Overhead Projector. This allows the instructor to face the class for better control of the learning situation. Materials may be prepared before showing. Line drawings on sheets of transparent material are used. The light is shown through the page and projected onto a screen. It is well adapted to dental health teaching since the instructor can use a previously illustrated tooth, have a class discussion and label the parts of the tooth and its supporting tissues. Thus, information and review are combined in one presentation.

Educational Television—Closed Circuit

Closed circuit television is one of the best media for team teaching. While subject matter is being explained and demonstrated by the special teacher, the classroom teacher is in the room to assist students in understanding the material presented. If several different classes have projectors they can all tune in to one lecture or demonstration. For those dental health teachers who aspire to become closed circuit television teachers the following attributes are pertinent: ability to teach in a classroom; competence in subject matter; creative and imaginative mind; ability to plan and develop a lesson and a course of study; ability to think and plan visually; a warm relaxed personality, a sense of humor; a cooperative attitude, with ability to take criticism; ability to communicate in a stimulating manner; ability to adjust to unexpected situations.

The studio teacher must communicate with the classroom teachers before each lesson. The communication is usually by means of a guide sheet which includes: points to be covered; list of facts to be learned for background; questions for discussion; key words; recommended books and reading sources.

The classroom teacher's responsibility is to relate the television presentation to the work being done in class. A discussion should follow the program, preferably right after the program has been presented. The teacher must note class reaction and stress habit and attitude changes as the desired outcome of the television presentation. Students should make an outline of the high points of the program.

Records and Tape Recordings

These media can be used for individual learning or amplified for group instruction. As a group activity it is not very effective in dental health instruction because it fails to hold attention for any length of time unless it is accompanied by some form of visual aid.

The slow learner can use a record and earphones and replay the record to learn the information at his own pace. Tape recordings serve as a means of preserving lessons in dental health for future use by classroom teachers. Recordings are also used as training devices. A playback will tend to clarify and correct information when preparing material for lectures. A recording will help to make corrections in pronunciation, diction and presentation. The difficulty of obtaining equipment, the cost and fragility of tapes and records make this medium less desirable than others.

Questions for Review and Discussion

In order to derive the most benefit from the following quiz, answers should be substantiated by statements from the text. Mark the following statements true(T) or false (F).

_____ 1. Health teaching has become functional, based on the needs and interests of children; therefore, little factual information is needed.

_____ 2. There is a complete transfer of knowledge to habit formation by exposing children to a good dental health film.

_____ 3. Since films, television and discussion groups have become popular there is little need for the traditional lecture.

_____ 4. Pretesting and post-testing are means by which the effectiveness of a television program can be measured.

_____ 5. Experimentation is the basis of learning.

_____ 6. Factual material is effectively learned if it is presented before showing a film.

_____ 7. No specific requirements are needed for team teaching other than knowing the subject.

_____ 8. Films and closed circuit television are economical because they require little preparation on the part of the classroom teacher.

_____ 9. One of the disadvantages of using posters in teaching is their scarcity.

_____ 10. Bulletin boards and exhibits may

remain in the school library indefinitely.

_____ 11. The use of the overhead and opaque projectors has many advantages over use of the chalkboard in teaching dental health.

_____ 12. Opaque and overhead projectors use the same materials.

Selected Readings

Anderson, C. L.: SCHOOL HEALTH PRACTICE, C. V. Mosby Co., St. Louis, 4th Edition, 1968, p. 237.

Audio-Visual Communication Review, Department of Audio-Visual Instruction, National Education Association, 1201 Sixteenth St., N. W., Washington, D. C. 20036. A periodical of teaching aids.

Brown, J. W., Lewis, R. B., Harclerood, F. F.: AUDIOVISUAL INSTRUCTION, McGraw-Hill, New York, 3rd Edition, 1969.

Dale, E.: AUDIO-VISUAL METHODS IN TEACHING, Dryden Press, New York, Revised Edition, 1954.

Davidson, R. L.: AUDIOVISUAL MACHINES, International Textbook Co., Scranton, Pa., 2nd Edition, 1969.

Nemir, A.: SCHOOL HEALTH PROGRAM, Appendix A—Resources, W. B. Saunders Co., Philadelphia, 3rd Edition, 1970.

Thomas, R. M., Swartout, S. G.: INTEGRATED TEACHING MATERIALS, David McKay Company, New York, 1963.

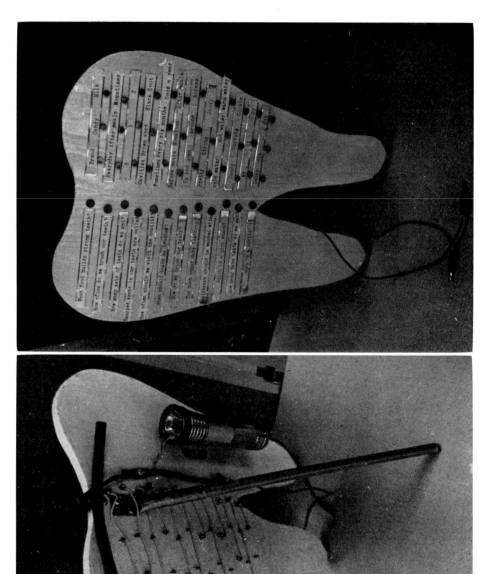

FIG. 28.—Creativity in producing visual aids adds interest to dental health teaching. The electrically operated question and answer board was produced by Gertrude Yarock, dental hygiene teacher, Tarrytown, New York, for use in the public schools.

Chapter 15

Group Activities and Interactions in Dental Health

Words are the medium of exchange of ideas between two or more persons wishing to communicate. They are spoken and heard or they are written and read. They stimulate and generate spontaneous response. They are a medium of free expression. Words are the keynote of giving and receiving information in all the situations to be discussed in this chapter.

Buzz Sessions or Small Group Discussion

The most informal form of communication is the buzz session or small group discussion. It provides for considerable interaction by students and allows free expression of ideas. If an idea is challenged, it should be accepted without criticism, recorded and later, in the discussion review, accepted or rejected. A good buzz session depends on a background of information. This form of communication is used in high school teaching.

It is difficult to control buzz sessions unless students are aware that a few may try to dominate the session. The teacher or student leader must keep the subject under discussion from being sidetracked by unrelated topics. Buzz sessions are most fruitful when students are motivated to continue their interest into an activity beyond the buzz session, for example, when they try to do something about the dental health problems of the community.

Class Discussions—Large Group Activity

Discussions following the presentation of new ideas in dental health are fruitful in bringing out the important points and in crystallizing the thinking of the group. As in buzz sessions, each person should be heard if he has anything to say and no ridicule or argumentation should be permitted. The whole group should be involved but everyone does not have to participate. If the discussions involve only a few students, the others become disinterested and bored. Class discussions are valuable instruments of learning when they are conducted on a background of information. All class discussions should have either a student or teacher as leader.

Panel Discussions

Panels are usually composed of three to five members, one of whom is the leader. The size of the panel will depend largely on the amount of time allotted to the discussion. One specific topic is investigated in depth. The panel may consist of experts or students or a mixture of both. Panels are conducted in an organized manner in contrast to an open discussion, as follows:

1. Each panel member prepares a five-to-ten minute talk during which he presents his point of view.

2. Each member has another five minutes for a rebuttal, which is usually his argu-

145

ment against another member's point of view.

3. At this point, the audience may be asked to enter into the discussion by asking pertinent questions.

4. The leader then sums up the arguments presented and makes recommendations for solving the problem.

5. The audience may infrequently enter into the decision by taking a vote from the floor. Decisions may be presented to the principal for consideration, acceptance or rejection, and action.

Discussion Leadership

The old idea that the leader is the authority has been abandoned in favor of the leader as a resource person; the one who provides the atmosphere of congenial thinking; the one who starts the conversation and then releases the flow of discussion to the other members of the group. The leader is considered a member of the group with special responsibilities. These are:

1. To control the other members, releasing creative thinking and suppressing the overtalkative.

2. To direct group thinking subtly, never dictatorially.

3. To help the group in setting goals, keep track of schedules and stop the discussion before the members are fatigued.

4. To correlate all proceedings, prevent emotional tensions, and smooth the way to objective thinking.

5. To be responsible for keeping the group working on the problem and headed toward a feasible solution. Good leadership comes with practice. The techniques of leadership should be studied and applied in all discussions.

Responsibilities of Members of a Discussion Group

The real strength of group action lies in the contributions of its individual members and the agreement that emerges in the form of decisions and actions. To this end each member has the responsibility of being an informed participant. If important decisions are to be made, learn as much as possible about all angles of the problem. Open-mindedness is the key to cooperation. Do not be afraid to change your mind, even though you have already expressed an opinion. In no case should you remain neutral or no action will take place. Read all communications before the meeting. Try to keep your thoughts focused on the main issues. Think objectively without being impersonal. Express dissent only when it has constructive value in coming to decisions. Show enthusiasm but keep your sense of humor under control.

Lectures

A lecture is a discourse on one particular subject delivered by one person. It is used extensively in college courses, but in elementary and high school the lecture is not really synonymous with teaching.

A good lecture should have an opening statement which gives the main theme. It should be expressed in such a way that it receives immediate attention but it should not be more than two or three short sentences.

The main value of a lecture is that a number of facts and concepts can be presented in a short time to a large number of people. There is no student participation and very little opportunity for creative thinking, except perhaps in the discussion following the lecture. Usually, there is no interaction between lecturer and learners. Lecturing requires exceptional knowledge of the subject as well as speaking skill. The lecturer must have enthusiasm for his subject and he must communicate this enthusiasm to the learners.

The following suggestions will assist in preparing and giving a lecture.

1. Prepare the oral presentation in detail on the basis of a definite purpose and expected outcomes.

2. Limit the number of facts presented and illustrate with examples and visual aids.

3. Adapt the lecture to the understanding as well as the interest of the group.

4. Give only specific and constructive details and express them clearly.

5. Be accurate in presenting dental health facts.

6. Use repetition in the summation to emphasize your main points.

7. Hold audience attention by using a pleasant voice and good sentence structure.

Field Trips

Dental health programs can provide a number of interesting field trips for learning by direct experience. A valuable learning experience for kindergarten or first-grade children results when the class goes to the school dental health room in preparation for the dental inspection. Elementary grades can have exciting and worthwhile experiences by visiting a free clinic or a dental office (many children have never seen one). A trip to a manufacturing plant where toothbrushes and dental instruments are made or to a plant where dentifrices and mouth washes are manufactured can be stimulating and educative for junior high school students.

Preplanning is indicated particularly when children are to leave the school grounds. Full responsibility for the safe conduct and return of the children to school must be assumed by the teacher. All rules and regulations made by the school board pertaining to parent consent slips, vehicles for travel and time schedules for leaving and returning to school must be kept. Parents' consent should always be in writing, as indicated in figure 29.

Pupils should participate in planning the trip as follows: a, determine what they are to look for during the trip; b, understand how the trip will help them to understand the problem being studied; c, understand that the trip will be pleasant but is primarily for the purpose of learning through observation; d, recognize the teacher's authority and be willing to abide by the rules of the trip.

Forms of Dramatic Experiences in Dental Health

Puppets. Dental health presents many opportunities for children to dramatize. All those experiences which allow the learner opportunities for role playing are included

---

THE WILLIAM JONES SCHOOL
Fairview, N.Y.

Date _____

Dear Parent or Guardian:

The _____ grade has planned an educational trip to _____

_____

on _____, by _____
　　　　　　month,　　day,　　year　　　　　　　　(name of transportation used)

The purpose of the field trip is to _____

The class will leave at _____ o'clock and return to school at _____. Kindly

give your permission for _____
　　　　　　　　　　　　　　　　　　　(name of the pupil)

_____

to accompany the class by signing below.

Sincerely yours,

(signed by the Principal or Teacher)

Parent's or Guardian's signature _____

FIG. 29.—Accepted form of permission and consent slip for field trips.

under the title of dramatic experiences. Puppet shows were among the earliest forms of theater and still appeal to children because of the humor of the puppet form and the size, which is more childlike than other types of dramatic art. Puppets are the little folks of imagination with whom the child can identify. The making of puppets is an art, but many dolls and playthings that children know and love become puppets in the hands of a skilled teacher. Puppetry is a form of lecture, with words and actions to convey facts and ideas of dental health. A small child believes puppets are real people. He carries away from a performance a lasting impression of what the puppets did and said.

Sociodrama or Role-playing. Sociodrama and role-playing are other forms of dramatic experiences. These are used principally to allow children free expression. The therapeutic value of emotional release through self-expression is well known. There are many instances where children can release tensions built up by dental ill health or fear of dental treatment.

Acting out the manner in which a tooth was injured at a drinking fountain in school is an excellent way of teaching accident prevention without preaching. Role-playing will frequently bring out the timid child, stimulating him to participate in group activities. While role-playing is unrehearsed and to a degree spontaneous, it is necessary for the teacher to have some control of the situation in order that positive attitudes are formed by the group.

Prepared Dramatizations versus Pupil-created Productions

There has been much controversy among educators as to the value of professionally written plays for health teaching. There appear to be more arguments for than against creative play in school situations. Dental health is so personal that many life situations contribute dramatic episodes. Consider the discomforts of poor dental health; the joy of a healthy mouth and a

good set of teeth; the exhilarating effect of—"Bobby, your treatment is all completed!"

Steps in Producing a Dental Health Assembly Program

To correlate dental health instruction with school activities, a dental health dramatization may be given as an assembly program. A playlet produced during National Dental Health Week, the first week in February, would be appropriate. Parents need instruction in dental health for their children, so they may be invited to attend. The first- or second-grade children may be chosen to present the playlet because this group will interest the greatest number of parents. Parents of first-grade children are most interested and eager to learn about their children's school experiences. They are receptive to dental health instruction.

1. The creation of a dental health play should be based on knowledge. Children should learn dental health facts before preparing the play so that they will have a body of knowledge upon which they may draw for the second step.

2. Several periods of discussion are scheduled for teacher and pupils to consider: a, What shall we name the play? (Naming the play may come at the end of the discussions if no conclusion is reached before the story is created.) b, Who are the people in the play? c, What will they do? Form an outline of the story. d, What will they say? Write the story. e, Try out several children for each part. Let the children decide who is best to play the part. f, Provide some opportunity for all children to participate in various ways such as a group scene, a marching scene, etc.

3. Preparation of props for the play: The children should make as many of the props as time and ability allow. Simplicity will add to the charm of the production. Less able children may operate the curtain, move the scenery and operate the lights. Consider the cost before entering upon elaborate stage settings.

4. Costuming: Parents like to have a part

in this phase of a school program. They will usually bear the cost and give more time to preparing costumes than teachers can give.

5. Rehearsals: Concentrated rehearsals just before the production is given are better than long, drawn-out rehearsals, as interest tends to lag. Give special sessions for the principal characters so as to prevent a discipline problem when children must wait around without activities.

6. Prepare invitations: The invitations should be handmade by the children and taken home to the parents several days before the assembly is scheduled.

7. Parents' conference: Allow sufficient time after the assembly for the parents to discuss dental health problems with the dentist or dental hygienist. A visit to the dental health room may be part of the conference.

8. Cooperation with special teachers: Dental health teachers should not attempt an assembly program that involves children without the full cooperation of the classroom teacher. If the art teacher and the music teacher are to be involved in the production, they should be notified well in advance of the time when their services will be needed. Each teacher has a heavy schedule. Be considerate in asking for time.

Questions for Review and Discussion

1. Describe the attributes of a good discussion leader.

2. Set up a vicarious situation in which one dental health problem is considered by a discussion group. Write out the arguments offered, pro and con. Present them as the leader of the group.

3. Pretend that you have a heckler in a group discussion. What means would you use to quiet him and convince him that the problem is serious and needs a solution?

4. "A man convinced against his will is of the same opinion still." List some means by which a person who resists changing his opinion might be convinced that the suggested changes will be beneficial for the dental health of school children.

5. Explain why group discussions are "in keeping with the principles of democratic action."

6. What are the responsibilities of members of a discussion group?

7. What is the principal difference between a discussion group and a buzz session?

8. Why is preplanning necessary before a field trip?

9. How would you explain "self-discipline" to a high school group during a planning session for a field trip?

10. How would you convince a parent that a field trip is educative and worthwhile?

Selected Readings

Anderson, R.: "How to Teach Better Listening," National Education Association Instructional Service, 1962.

Beggs, D. W.: TEAM TEACHING, Indiana University Press, Bloomington, Indiana, 4th Edition, 1967.

Borman, E. G.: DISCUSSION AND GROUP METHODS, Harper & Row, New York, 1969.

Bye, E. C.: "How to Conduct a Field Trip," National Council for the Social Studies, National Education Association.

Dickinson, M. B.: "Independent and Group Learning," Elementary Instructional Service, National Education Association.

Fodor, J. T., Dalis, G. T.: HEALTH INSTRUCTION: THEORY AND APPLICATION, Lea & Febiger, Philadelphia, 1966, p. 82.

Schatz, E.: "The Teacher as a Learner," National Education Association Instructional Service, 1962.

Zeleny, D. L.: "How to Use Sociodrama," National Council for the Social Studies, National Education Association.

APPENDIX

The Growth and Functions of the Mouth and the Teeth

Knowledge of the anatomy and physiology of the human mouth and teeth is important to all those who teach dental health. Those who have scientific knowledge of these parts should be able to instruct children and adults in simple, understandable terms. *This appendix may seem to be oversimplified in order to fulfill these purposes.* The appendix may also help teachers to prepare lesson plans, lectures and other educative media without having to do extensive research.

Basic understanding should include knowledge of the mechanism of mastication; the normal range of eruption dates for both the primary (deciduous) and the permanent set of teeth (dentition). An understanding of normal occlusion will provide the dental educator with information so that deviations from the normal may be detected and brought to the attention of parents. The teeth, the jaws and the mouth should be considered as integral parts of the entire body. Any condition which affects the growth and development of the body is apt to affect the formation, calcification and the alignment of the teeth in the dental arches.

The Head

At birth the skull is large in proportion to other parts of the skeleton, but the facial portion is small due to the incomplete development of the upper and lower jaws and maxillary sinuses. It is only equal to about one-eighth of the bulk of the cranium. The adult face equals about one-half of the cranium. Calcification of the bones of the head is not complete at birth. Many bones are still partly cartilage. For example, the hard palate (the roof of the mouth) is not completely calcified at the midline.

Because the face is small at birth rapid growth takes place during the first years of life. Unfavorable influences may alter the development to quite a marked degree. Improper sleeping habits, improper use of nursing bottles, too short or too long periods of nursing and prolonged habits of sucking of thumb, finger, lip and tongue are undesirable and can have marked influence on the development and changing structures of the face and mouth. The future shape and formation of the child's face are determined by the growth and development of the teeth and jaws. The development of the jaws is in a state of continuing growth, more so than the rest of the skull. Great care and watchfulness are necessary so that children do not acquire abnormal habits that affect the normal symmetry of the face and jaws.

The jaws are formed during the eighth to tenth week of fetal life. The upper jaw is formed of the two maxillary bones and the palatine bones and it is known as the

151

maxilla. Before birth these bones usually unite to form the hard palate or the roof of the mouth. Failure of these parts to unite results in cleft palate and lip.

There are several sinuses or hollow chambers within the maxilla. Among them are the maxillary sinuses located above the upper molar and bicuspid teeth. Abnormal conditions of the nose and diseased conditions of the teeth may cause infections in these sinuses, a serious health impairment.

The lower jaw is known as the *mandible.* It is the strongest bone in the face. At birth it consists of two parts which grow together to form one bone at the midline of the face during the first and second year of life. Beginning of ossifications of the lower jaw takes place about the sixth week of fetal life. It resembles a horseshoe in form. The vertical portion of the mandible ends in a saddle shape which forms the joint with the temporal bone. The mandible is the only movable bone in the head. It has no bony union with the skull but depends on muscles and ligaments to hold it in place. The joint where the mandible and the maxilla meet is called the temporomandibular joint. Each jaw supports ten teeth of the primary set and later sixteen teeth of the permanent set.

The Mechanism of Mastication

Thinking in the past of dental care for children was geared to a life expectancy of 30 to 35 years. Now the long-range concern for dental health extends to a life expectancy of 65 years of age or longer. It is apparent then that the need for maintaining a good vitality and a good reserve capacity is important. It is the responsibility of all concerned with health to give guidance early in the life of the child so that he will develop and maintain ability to chew his food throughout his expected life span.

The child poses many problems of growth and development both physical and mental. If guidance is to be effective, the *function* of teeth must be taught in relation to their structure. While it is necessary to avoid

dental infection, it is equally important to maintain good chewing function.

The infant instinctively bites and attempts to chew. The child, however, does not learn to use his chewing mechanism until he has all his primary teeth and has had time to develop efficiency in using them. This takes about the first three years of life. In fact, the child must be taught to chew, just as he is taught to walk or speak. In order to chew effectively the child must learn the following:

1. to control his lower jaw
2. to control the tongue from the backward-and-forward movement in sucking to the side-to-side movement in chewing
3. to coordinate the muscles of the tongue and cheeks so that food is held for chewing between the upper and lower back teeth
4. how long to chew before swallowing food
5. to close lips and to force the food back into the throat to keep food from dribbling out of the mouth during swallowing
6. to accept larger particles of food and harder foods gradually, so that the teeth and jaws will be exercised and will develop.

What is frequently thought to be lack of appetite in small children has been traced to pain or discomfort of the teeth and undue effort in chewing. The child with impaired chewing function is crippled; he will tend to eat only those foods which he can chew comfortably. A number of undesirable swallowing habits as well as tongue and lip habits can be traced to improper use of the chewing mechanism. Therefore, proper use of the teeth, lips, tongue and jaws during mastication must be part of all dental health instruction.

Many young children ask, "How do I chew?" Few of them realize that in chewing only their lower jaw moves. The mandible moves in a number of directions during the process of chewing. In order to chew properly a whole system of parts in the head and mouth come into play. These parts are called the *masticatory system.* It is composed of the teeth and their supporting parts, the jaws, the temporomandibular joint, the muscles attached to the lower jaw, the lips and the tongue, the blood vessels and the nerves that supply these parts. In addition to these parts we might add the salivary glands which excrete saliva that lubricates and partially digests the food. All these are capable of acting as a unit not only for the purpose of chewing, but also for sucking, speaking and expressing certain emotions. Chewing is the first step in food digestion. It is known that people who do not chew properly fail to digest considerable amounts of food, especially meats and vegetables that are tough and fibrous.

The action of breaking up food takes place on the surface of the teeth as they meet each other in a number of positions. These actions take place mainly on the molar teeth although the bicuspids enter into the action of chewing and also direct the food back to the molars. Chewing is primarily a rotary movement of the mandible, with a cutting thrust as the teeth come together in normal position. During the cycle of chewing there is a momentary crushing as the lower molars act on the upper molars in an action similar to the crushing action of a mortar and pestle. Figure 30 shows the three positions of the upper and lower molars during the chewing cycle. It explains how teeth that are formed with high cusps and deep grooves are able to function. It also indicates how the loss of even one tooth destroys the exact pattern of mastication.

The Development of the Teeth

During the sixth week of fetal life growth changes take place in each of the three primary layers which form the human body. The outer layer, called the ectoderm, forms twenty tooth buds, ten in each jaw. These buds become the enamel organs and in them grow the twenty primary or first teeth. When the tooth grows into its chewing position in the mouth, a very thin layer of the enamel organ remains on the tooth. It is sometimes referred to as the skin of the tooth. It is worn off by the action of chewing, toothbrushing and other types of attrition to which the tooth is subject.

The permanent teeth develop in much the same way, except that the enamel

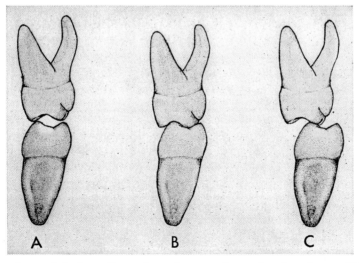

FIG. 30.—*A*, The relation of the lower first molar to the upper first molar when the mandible closes on the maxilla. *B*, The centric relationship in which the mortar and pestle action takes place. *C*, The lower molar moves to the side and pushes the food in that direction as the mandible drops away in preparation for a second cycle of the chewing action. (From Wheeler, *Textbook of Dental Anatomy and Physiology*, courtesy, W. B. Saunders Co.)

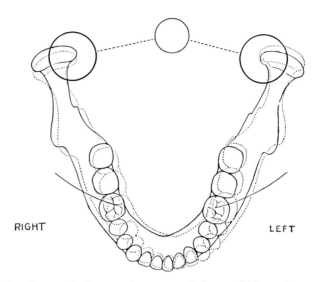

FIG. 31.—A tracing of a photograph showing the motion of the mandible in the action of chewing. The heavy line shows the mandible in central position. Dotted line shows movement to the left. Similar movement takes place to the front and to the right, completing the cycle. All movements occur within the area indicated by the circles at the joint (temporomandibular joint). (From Wheeler, *Textbook of Dental Anatomy and Physiology,* courtesy, W. B. Saunders Co.)

organs of the permanent teeth develop as a budding process branching off from the enamel organ of the primary teeth to form the thirty-two teeth of the permanent set. Only the first permanent molars (sixth year molars) of the permanent set show the beginning of growth at birth. All the other permanent teeth develop after birth. Therefore, they are affected by the general health of the child during the first eight years of life.

During this growth process each tooth develops a shape and size according to its position and use. Each jaw may be divided into two equal parts, the right and the left sides. For the purpose of discussion we may say that each portion has five primary teeth. Counting from the midline they are as follows:

1. Central incisor ⎱ sharp, chisel-shaped teeth
2. Lateral incisor ⎰ used for cutting food.
3. Cuspid—a pointed tooth used for grasping and tearing.
4. First primary molar ⎱ broad flat chewing
5. Second primary molar ⎰ surfaces for grinding food.

There are thirty-two teeth in the permanent set (dentition):

1. Central incisor
2. Lateral incisor
3. Cuspid
4. First bicuspid
5. Second bicuspid
6. First permanent molar
7. Second permanent molar
8. Third permanent molar

The increase in number of permanent teeth over the primary set is accounted for by the three permanent molars which erupt behind the primary molars. The primary molars are replaced by the bicuspid teeth. These are the only "new teeth" as far as function is concerned. They partially crush food and direct it backward to be ground by the molars. The incisors and cuspids are referred to as anterior or front teeth; the bicuspids and molars as posterior or back teeth.

Eruption of Teeth

The normal physiological process by which the crown of a tooth breaks through the bone and gum tissue and appears in the mouth is called eruption of a tooth. The time of eruption of the primary and the permanent teeth varies with each individual

THE DECIDUOUS (PRIMARY) TEETH

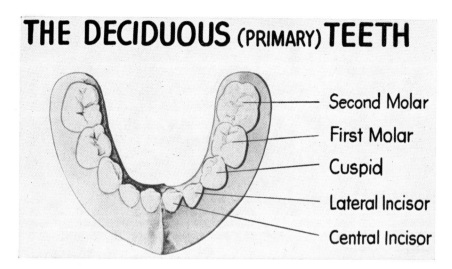

- Second Molar
- First Molar
- Cuspid
- Lateral Incisor
- Central Incisor

THE PERMANENT TEETH

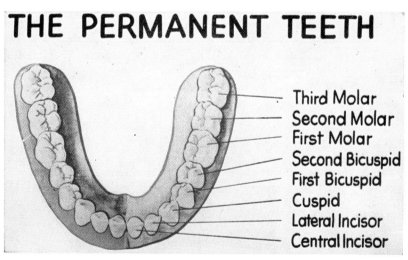

- Third Molar
- Second Molar
- First Molar
- Second Bicuspid
- First Bicuspid
- Cuspid
- Lateral Incisor
- Central Incisor

Fig. 32.—Diagrammatic arrangement of teeth in the lower jaw. (Courtesy, *The American Dental Association.*)

child and has no bearing on the future resistance of the tooth to decay. Although all of the factors associated with tooth eruption are not known, it is thought that the growth of the jaws and the growth of the root are important factors.

As the crown develops it lies in a bony crypt within the jaw bone. As the development of the tooth progresses the pressure exerted by the growing crown causes the bone above it to resorb (a gradual breaking down and dissolving of the bone). At the same time the root of the tooth grows longer and the bone grows in layers at the end (apex) of the root. Both activities produce pressure on the soft tissue (the gum) and the blood supply in it is cut off; the tissue above the tooth becames thin, and finally perforates, allowing the tip of the crown to show in the mouth. The process of eruption continues until the crown of the tooth meets its opposing tooth or teeth in the opposite jaw. During this time the root continues to grow until its form is completed and the apex nearly closes, leaving a small opening sufficient to allow the blood

Table 12.—Approximate Eruption Dates of Primary Teeth

Teeth of the upper jaw (maxilla)	Central incisor	7½	months	of	age
	Lateral incisor	9	"	"	"
	Cuspid	18	"	"	"
	First molar	14	"	"	"
	Second molar	24	"	"	"
Teeth of the lower jaw (mandible)	Central incisor	6	"	"	"
	Lateral incisor	7	"	"	"
	Cuspid	16	"	"	"
	First molar	12	"	"	"
	Second molar	20	"	"	"

Approximate Eruption Dates of Permanent Teeth

Central incisor	7–8	years	of	age
Lateral incisor	8–9	"	"	"
Cuspid	11–12	"	"	"
First bicuspid	10–11	"	"	"
Second bicuspid	10–12	"	"	"
First molar	6–7	"	"	"
Second molar	11–13	"	"	"
Third molar	17–21	"	"	"

(Adapted from Orban after Logan and Kronfeld [slightly modified by McCall and Schour] as reported in *Oral Embryology and Microscopic Anatomy* by Permar, 4th Edition, Lea & Febiger, 1967.)

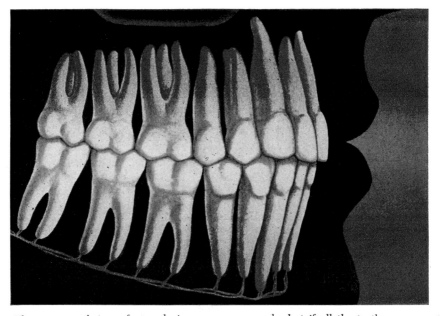

FIG. 33.—Thirty-two teeth in perfect occlusion occur very rarely, but if all the teeth are present in the mouth and malocclusion is negligible there will be equal pressure during mastication, which tends to exercise the teeth and to build stronger supporting structures.

vessels and nerves to pass through so that they may nourish the pulp of the tooth.

The First Permanent Molar

This tooth has been called the most important tooth in the permanent set. The four first permanent molars provide the means of stabilizing the position of the two jaws in relation to each other during the time when the primary teeth are being shed. They form a guide for the alignment of the permanent teeth as they erupt.

The first permanent molar is the sixth tooth from the midline of the jaw in both the primary and permanent set. It usually erupts about the sixth year of life and has therefore been called the "sixth year molar." It erupts before the primary teeth are shed. It does not replace a primary tooth. Therefore it is frequently mistaken for a primary tooth. It is subject to dental decay early in life; it is neglected and frequently extracted. If the first permanent molars are lost early in life, the entire arch will suffer loss of balance and will eventually show malocclusion.

Parts of the Tooth

Each tooth has a crown and a root portion. The crown is covered with *enamel* and the root is covered with *cementum*. The bulk of the tooth is composed of dentin. These are the hard or calcified tissues of the tooth. They are composed primarily of the same materials, principally calcium and phosphorus salts, with varying amounts of organic material. The composition of these calcified tissues varies in density, thickness and structure. The teeth have five functions, (1) to masticate food, (2) to afford proper speech, (3) to aid appearance, (4) to assist digestion of food and (5) to give shape to the face.

There is also a soft tissue contained in a chamber within the dentin and leading from the tooth through a small channel or canal through each root. It is called the tooth pulp.

The *enamel* is the outer covering of the crown of the tooth which is seen in the mouth. It is smooth and hard so as to resist the strain and the wear of chewing. It also protects the softer dentin underneath.

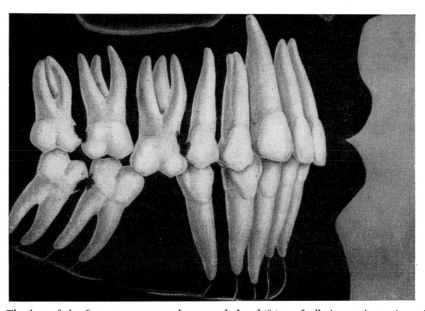

FIG. 34.—The loss of the first permanent molar caused the shifting of all the teeth on this side of the mouth. The upper first molar has grown down to meet the second bicuspid and the second molar of the lower jaw. Uneven pressure causes them to tilt and to lose contact with their adjacent teeth. Cavities develop between the teeth. (Courtesy, *The American Dental Association.*)

Enamel is considered the hardest tissue in the body. It is quite brittle since it contains very little organic material in its structure. Hard objects should not be cut, crushed or broken by the teeth because its enamel, which is made of tiny rods, will split apart and cause a break in the tooth. The enamel cannot repair itself as do other body tissues. Therefore any break in the enamel must be repaired by the dentist.

The *dentin* forms the bulk of the entire tooth. It contains more organic matter than the enamel because there are many canals running through it which bring nourishment from the dental pulp. The dentin gives elasticity to the tooth so that during mastication the pressure will not break the tooth apart.

The *cementum* is a modified form of bone which is arranged in thin layers around the root of the tooth. It is thin near the enamel border and becomes thicker toward the end (apex) of the root. Its chief function is to form a suitable surface to which the soft fibers from the membrane surrounding the tooth in its socket (periodontal membrane) may attach. These fibers are also attached to the jaw bone, thus holding the tooth firmly in the socket so that it can function for chewing.

The *pulp* of the tooth is composed of blood vessels and nerve fibers held together by connective tissue in the pulp chamber. The function of the pulp is to provide nourishment and sensation to the tooth. The nerve fibers in the pulp communicate pain to the brain when a cavity becomes large. The blood vessels and nerves of the pulp

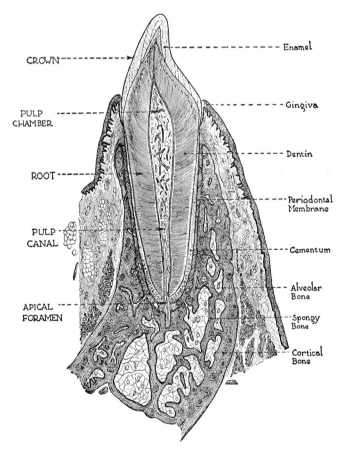

Fig. 35.—Diagrammatic representation of the dental tissues. (Schour, *Noyes' Oral Histology and Embryology*, Lea & Febiger, 1960.)

lead out of the tooth through the root canal and join with the blood vessels and the nerve fibers in the jaws.

Structures That Support the Teeth in the Mouth

The *periodontal membrane* is a delicate tissue which surrounds the tooth in its socket. It is composed of many types of cells which have special functions, namely, *a,* to form the cementum which covers the root of the tooth; *b,* to form fibers which attach to the bone of the tooth socket; *c,* to form fibers which attach to the cementum of the root.

The periodontal membrane has several other functions: *a,* It supports the tooth in its socket by the series of fibers which resist lateral and horizontal pressures. The fibers at the end of the root resist the forces that tend to lift the tooth from its socket or tilt it from side to side. If the periodontal membrane is seriously injured, the tooth becomes loose. *b,* The formative function of the periodontal membrane includes tooth development before eruption; the formation of cementum and the bone of the tooth socket. It continues to form cementum and bone throughout the life of the tooth. *c,* The periodontal membrane also helps in the resorption and formation of bone. It is therefore possible to move teeth in their sockets in a desired direction and to build bone on the opposite side to hold the tooth in the new position. Orthodontists take advantage of this natural process in straightening teeth.

The *alveolar process* is that part of the jaw bone which forms the socket of the tooth. It is a very thin layer of bone and is easily destroyed by undue pressure or infection. The alveolar bone will regenerate if the traumatic action and infection are removed. It is covered by the gum (the gingiva). The health of this thin plate of bone which surrounds each tooth depends in a large measure on the proper alignment of the teeth in the upper jaw in relation to the teeth of the lower jaw. The degeneration of the alveolar process due to infection and uneven stress on the teeth during mastication results in the loss of a great number of teeth in later life.

The *gingiva* is that part of the lining of the mouth which covers the alveolar bone and surrounds each tooth. It also forms the small points of tissue (papillae) seen between teeth. The gingiva is continuous with the periodontal membrane. In appearance normal gingiva is light pink; has a stippled appearance and is securely attached to the underlying tissues. The gingiva is tougher than other parts of the lining of the mouth so that it can withstand all the stresses of mastication. The more it is used the stronger it becomes.

The *mucosa* or the lining of the mouth is a mucous membrane which is similar in structure to the linings of other body cavities that open to the outside such as the stomach, the intestine and the bronchi leading to the lungs. The lining of the cheeks, lips and the area under the tongue is covered with this soft, red tissue which contains many blood and lymph vessels as well as the mucus-producing glands. Although it is easily injured, the mucosa has great ability to repair and regenerate.

Saliva is a fluid that is produced by the salivary glands. It is discharged into the mouth through ducts and acts as a lubricant for all the mouth structures. Saliva has a definite part in the process of mastication and digestion. It moistens the food so that it can be chewed and swallowed. It contains an enzyme (chemical that speeds up digestion) that begins the process of digestion of carbohydrates. The saliva also contains additional substances that act to prevent the mouth from becoming too acid or too alkaline. This is called the buffer action of saliva and aids in the prevention of dental decay. The saliva is one of nature's ways of cleaning the teeth by constantly bathing them in a fresh supply. The saliva also acts to inhibit the growth of certain bacteria which are harmful to health. About three pints of saliva are produced every day.

There are several sets of salivary glands in the mouth. Small glands are located on the tongue. The larger sets are located under the mucosa.

Parotid glands are located in front of and below each ear. Submaxillary glands are located on the inner surface of the lower jaw in front of the jaw angle. The sublingual glands are located beneath the tongue on the floor of the mouth.

Shedding the Primary Teeth (Exfoliation)

The roots of the primary teeth are completely formed two years after the teeth erupt into the mouth. During this time the crowns of the permanent teeth have been forming under the primary teeth roots. Gradually pressure is exerted by the growing permanent tooth upon the root of the primary tooth, causing the resorption of the primary root. When only a hollow crown remains attached to the gum tissue the primary crown falls out. Frequently this occurrence leads to the erroneous idea that primary teeth have no roots. Soon after the shedding of the primary tooth the permanent tooth appears.

This appendix is an attempt to simplify the complex structures and the growth processes of the mouth and teeth so that those who teach may learn to express these scientific facts in simple, understandable words.

Vocabulary Related to the Parts and Structures of the Teeth

1. BICUSPID—there are eight bicuspids, four in each jaw. The first and second bicuspids are found between the cuspids and molars. These teeth have two cusps, one or two roots, and are used to tear and grind food.
2. BLOOD VESSELS—the channels (arteries, veins or capillaries) through which blood flows to nourish the teeth.
3. CEMENTUM—a bonelike substance which covers the dentin of the tooth in the root area.
4. CROWN—the part of the tooth, covered with enamel, which, when it has erupted, is visible in the mouth.
5. CUSPID—there are four cuspids, two in each jaw and located in the corners of the mouth between the lateral incisors and first bicuspids. The crown of the cuspid is a single sharp projection or cusp, and there is one root. The cuspids are used for tearing food.
6. DENTAL CARIES—a localized disease that destroys tooth structure, producing cavities in the teeth. Dental caries is commonly called tooth decay.
7. DENTIN—an ivorylike substance, softer than the enamel, that forms the body of the tooth. It consists of a matrix containing minute parallel tubules which open into the pulp cavity and contain during life dentinal fibers of the cells of the pulp.
8. ENAMEL—the hard, white, outer covering of the crowns of the teeth. It is the hardest substance of the body. It consists of minute prisms arranged at right angles to the surface and bound together by a cement substance.
9. GUM— (The gingiva) the pink-colored tissue which surrounds the necks of teeth and covers the part of the jaws where the sockets for the teeth are situated.
10. INCISORS—central or first incisors—there are four central or first incisors, two in each jaw. They are the front center teeth in the mouth and are used to cut food. The crowns are flat and sharp and there is one root. Lateral or second incisors—there are four lateral or second incisors, two in each jaw, one next to each of the central incisors. The crowns of these teeth are also flat and sharp and the roots are single. The lateral incisors also serve to cut food.
11. JAWS—two bony structures in which the teeth are located.
12. MOLAR—there are twelve permanent molars in all. They are located to the rear of the bicuspids. Molars have several cusps; upper molars usually have three roots and the lower molars two. Permanent molars are not preceded by primary teeth. These teeth serve to grind food. The word "molar" comes from the Latin and French words meaning "mill."
13. NECK—a slightly narrowed portion of the tooth where the root and crown meet.
14. NERVES—cordlike bands of nervous tissue which connect the brain and spinal cord with other organs of the body, and conduct nervous impulses to or away from these organs.
15. PERMANENT TEETH—the second set of teeth which should last a lifetime, thirty-two in number.
16. PRIMARY TEETH—the first set of teeth, twenty in number.
17. PULP—the tissue located inside the tooth which contains the blood supply and which supplies sensation to the tooth.
18. ROOT—the part of the tooth by which it is attached in the socket of the jaw. The root is covered with cementum.
19. SIX-YEAR MOLAR—the first *permanent* molar. There are four—one on each half of each jaw. It should be the sixth tooth from the midline. It is not preceded by a primary tooth.
20. STRUCTURE—the arrangement of parts, particles and tissues into parts of a body.
21. WISDOM TOOTH—the third molar; the last teeth of the full permanent set on each half of each jaw of man, familiarly so called, because they appear when the person may be supposed to have acquired some wisdom.

Suggested Enriched Vocabulary

1. CALCIUM—a mineral; essential to the growth and health of bones and teeth.
2. CARBOHYDRATES—sugar and starch groups. Fermentable carbohydrates (principally sugars), plus the action of bacteria, cause dental caries.
3. DENTIFRICE—paste, powder or liquid used as a mechanical aid to the toothbrush in the act of cleansing the teeth.
4. DENTAL HYGIENIST—a trained person, usually a woman, who cleans teeth and instructs in the hygienic care of the teeth and mouth.
5. FLUORIDATION—adjustment of the fluoride content upward to a desirable level in water deficient in the substance.
6. GINGIVITIS—inflammation of the gums.
7. MALOCCLUSION—term applied to irregularities in the position of the teeth and the improper coming together of the teeth upon closing the jaws.
8. OCCLUSION—the bringing of the opposing surfaces of the teeth of the two jaws into contact; also, the relation between the surfaces of teeth when in contact.
9. ORTHODONTIST—a dentist who has had special training in and practices the diagnosis and treatment of irregularities of the teeth.
10. PERIODONTAL DISEASE—disease of any of the supporting structures of the teeth such as gums, periodontal membrane, bone.
11. PHOSPHORUS—a mineral essential to the growth and health of bones and teeth.
12. PROPHYLAXIS—measures directed to the prevention of diseases of the mouth; cleaning of the teeth by a dentist or dental hygienist.
13. X RAY (noun)—a photograph which penetrates the surface and reveals the inner parts of the teeth.
    X-RAY (adjective)
    X RAY (verb transitive)—to expose to the action of X rays; to examine, treat, or photograph, with X rays.

Index